A WOMAN'S RECIPE FOR LIFE

A Nurturing Approach
Throughout Womanhood
from Adolescence to Aging

Katy O'Neal Arrowood

This book is dedicated to

my entire family, but most especially,

my younger brother,

GLENN HAMILTON KEITH O'NEAL

who through his untimely death

at the age of 18,

taught me how precious and fragile life is.

We must all live each day to the fullest,

and be forever committed

to the service of others.

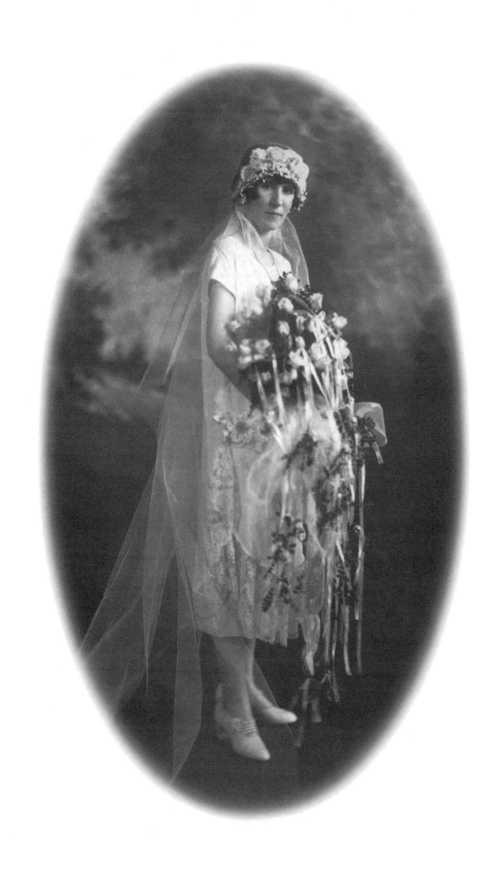

Acknowledgments

First, I would like to thank my husband, Ben, who has always encouraged me to be my best. Thanks to Keith, whose birth changed our lives, and who ultimately through his birth, inspired me to create my career, eventually leading to this book.

My parents, too, are at the top of the list. They have offered unconditional love and support throughout my life. I have gained so many blessings from them, I could never list them all.

Thanks to Dr. Reuben Smith, Dr. Robert Kelley, Dr. Leon Smith, Dr. Cynthia Mercer, Dr. Margaret Cramer, Dr. Anne Ford, and Betty Parker, RN, manager. It was through their vision that my career as a family management consultant was born. Thanks for giving me the freedom to find creative ways to meet the needs of your patients. With this position, and this book, you have truly given me the chance of a lifetime.

Appreciation is also expressed to the staff of Athens Women's Clinic. We are truly a support staff, offering support to both our patients and each other; it is their family photos that helped to complete this book.

The expertise of Lorena Akioka as editor, and Digital Impact as designers, helped to make this dream a reality. Don Bagwell, Max Harrell, and Sara Zimmerman Huber worked diligently as well as patiently, as the book began to unfold. Lorena proved herself very early on in the project. As a team, Lorena, Don, Max, and Sara are unbeatable.

Finally, thanks to all of the women with whom I have worked. I have learned from you far more than I could ever give. So to the many of you who have inspired me during various stages of my life, I dedicate this book.

COVER: Photograph of Bea Carter, Wendy Waites, and Elora Marable in the kitchen of Jim and Sue Carter (Madison, Georgia). Photography by David Greear, Digital Impact Design.

Introduction

I was born into a family of educators; many chose education as a career, others offered me invaluable lessons about life. Fortunately, I recorded many of these life lessons; some in the corners of my mind, many on scraps of paper. Often, I would find ways to offer support to others through my own experiences, as well as those of my family.

I am blessed to have extraordinary parents and caring siblings. They each give me so much. The most tragic event for my family was the death of my younger brother, Glenn. He died suddenly at the age of 18 due to a seizure disorder caused by a childhood head injury. At this point, grief was thrust upon me in a way I could never have imagined. His death still has such an impact on all of us; thankfully, the healing has begun.

One of the happiest days of my life brought with it a huge challenge. When I married Ben, I became a stepmother to Stephanie and Ashley. Although Ben did not have custody, he did have visitation rights. This began my bumpy road in seeking to be a supportive wife, as well as an effective step-parent.

One of my very best teachers was my grandmother, May Belle Odom Keith. Grandmama lived to be 92, and she remained a thriving, productive, and gracious woman until her life ended. She taught me to grow old gracefully.

Through my grandmother's life, and by watching and participating in my own mother's aging process, I have learned many things. Some of these experiences I have passed on to Athens Women's Clinic's menopause support group, in which I am the facilitator. By listening carefully and taking many notes, I have gleaned many hints from the many women who have participated in and been helped by this group.

I was extremely blessed during the pregnancy with my first child. I was remarkably healthy, the baby was thriving, and my husband and I were happy—what more could I ask? Then I realized that I had many other unanswered questions. How was I going to be an effective working mom? What would help me in encouraging my husband to stay involved in our dual career household? What about budgeting for our future as a family? How would my stepdaughters handle this new addition? And there were so many more questions.

Although I had a wonderful obstetrician, many of these questions were not addressed. He proficiently handled my medical needs, but I would need to go elsewhere for the non-medical needs. About 20 weeks into my pregnancy, I sat in his office and cried. I wanted more than just good medical care; I wanted some comforting answers to the other pressing concerns.

Keith Benedict Arrowood arrived on October 30, 1991. What an impact he made in our lives! Soon after his arrival, I decided to leave behind a restaurant/catering business and become a full-time mother. I relished the time I spent at home with Keith, but due to necessity, after a year, I planned to return to the work force. As a woman of the '90s, I decided to use my educational background in child and family development, as well as my own life experiences, to create a career. I remembered all of the non-medical questions I faced during my pregnancy, and thought: "Wouldn't it be great to be that resource person available to meet the non-medical needs of others?"

I met with several professionals in the field of human development and, ultimately, the position of a family management consultant was conceived. In order to be available to a large number of women, the most logical placement of this new position would be with a group of obstetricians/gynecologists..

I began to pursue a progressive group of physicians who were truly dedicated to the total care of women. Fortunately, my search ended quickly. Athens Women's Clinic saw the need for this resource, and my skills meshed perfectly with the thorough medical care they offered.

Through this position, I have met with thousands of women facing various challenges during distinct life stages. As with any newly created position, I knew the importance of keeping good records. Eventually, I had a collection of tips, suggestions, and resources that had proved helpful to many women, as well as being invaluable to me. This book includes that collection of useful advice.

As a woman, I also know the importance of food in our lives. We plan and produce meals for our families; we often coordinate gatherings—large and small—that involve food in some fashion; and as women we must practice healthy eating habits. I have always loved cooking for myself and for others. This joy of working with food was expressed through my restaurant and catering business, and is practiced daily within my own home. I have taken many of my favorite recipes and incorporated them into this book. (Most are low fat, some are sinful!) I have also included menu plans that have proven to be workable for Athens Women's Clinic's patients.

The suggestions, menus, and easy recipes included in this book have been a significant source of assistance to many women. I hope they will do the same for you.

Katy O'Neal Arrowood holds a degree in Family and Consumer Sciences, with an emphasis in child and family development from The University of Georgia. She is also a Certified Family Life Educator, as sponsored by the National Council on Family Relations.

Currently, Katy is the Family Management Consultant for Athens Women's Clinic, a position she created. She has appeared in various publications and is a regular guest on Atlanta's WXIA/Channel 11 Noonday program.

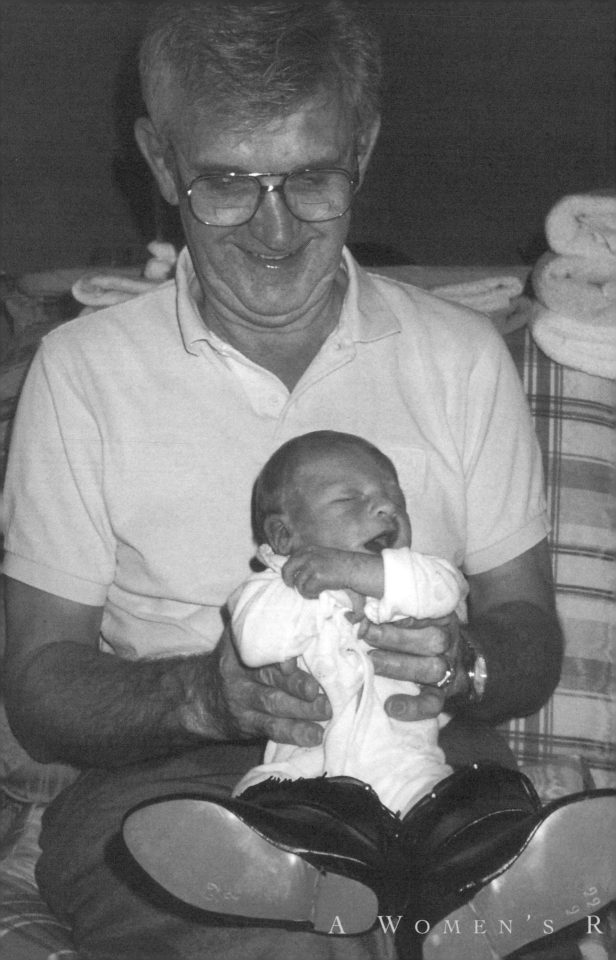

CONTENTS

Begi

nings

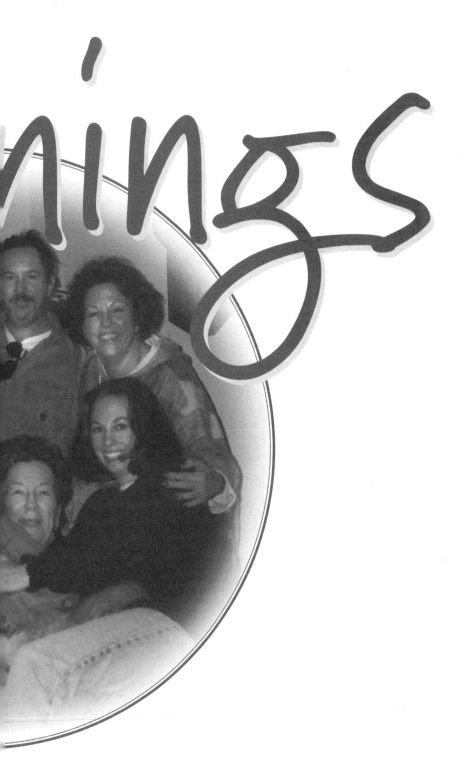

'Tis beauty
that doth oft
make women
proud;
'Tis virtue,
that doth make
them most
admired;
'Tis modesty,
that makes
them seem
divine.

— Shakespeare

2

Selecting Your Obstetrician/Gynecologist

As a woman, there is one decision that you will make that will affect your life during many of its milestones, a decision that will influence the quality of every-day living, as well as the way you view yourself. I am referring to your choice of a gynecologist. Due to circumstances, this decision may be made more than once in your lifetime, and each time you should make the most educated choice possible.

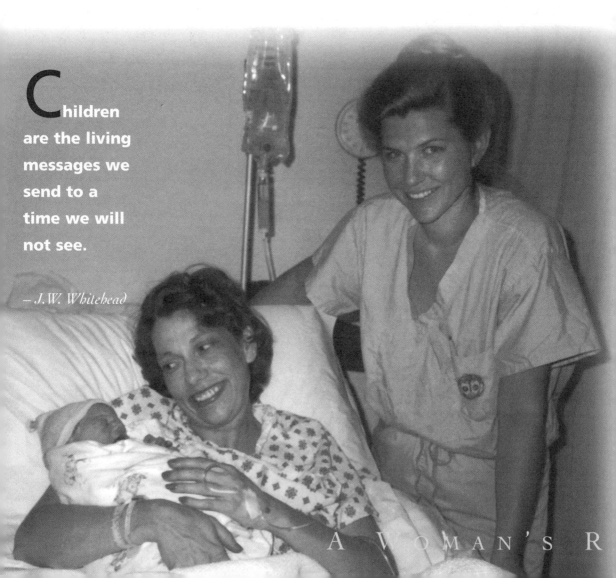

Children are the living messages we send to a time we will not see.

– J.W. Whitehead

Traditionally, women have used their obstetrician/gynecologist as a "catch all" physician, who assists in all facets of family planning, whether it is birth control options, pre-conception care, prenatal care, or infertility. This same physician will be there as you begin the aging process, including premenopausal symptoms, the onset of menopause, and your post-menopausal reality.

Your ob/gyn will provide your health care, but as most women know, a good ob/gyn also furnishes you with much more. From referrals to other professionals, to support and comfort during many of life's changes, your ob/gyn should play a significant part in your continuous emergence as a confidant, productive woman.

Your first appointment should be when you are 18 years old, or have become sexually active. You should see your ob/gyn once a year, except during pregnancy, infertility treatments, menopause, or any other event that warrants more visits. One portion of the selection process should include the type of medical practice you seek. There are solo practitioners, as well as partners, and groups of physicians. For your ob/gyn care, you will have one physician, whether in a solo practice or a group, who will be the primary provider, and who you will come to know very personally. The difference between solo practices and a group is more obvious during pregnancy.

"I want to see the same physician for all of my obstetrical visits," is the primary reason many women give for choosing a solo practitioner. This may be an advantage, but in reality, if this doctor is called to the hospital, appointments may be delayed or be rescheduled. Another concern is if your physician is out of town when you go into labor, a back-up physician, whom you may never have met will be substituted.

There are, however, many advantages to selecting a group of obstetrician/ gynecologists. Since you will see everyone in the group during your prenatal care, this assures that you will see a familiar face during labor. Another advantage is the opportunity for the physicians to consult as a group over a high-risk pregnancy, knowing that in may situations "two heads are better than one." One other advantage is the capability of a group to offer state-of-the-art equipment as well as other professionals within the practice to insure that all patients receive optimum care.

A safe way to begin your selection is to ask a close friend or family member for the name of her ob/gyn. As an adolescent, you may want to use your mother's physician or someone within the same group. Ask a lot of questions of others and be sure to include questions pertaining to your values and beliefs.

Once the list has been narrowed, call the offices in which you are most interested to find out more about the practice. Your initial reaction to the reception you get from this phone call will tell you about the office. Did they take the time to answer your questions or have someone call you back at a more convenient time; or do you feel that you are being a nuisance for calling? Find a practice that feels comfortable to you.

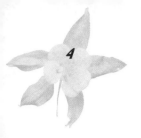

On your first visit to the physician, be sure that this person is someone you can trust; after all, she will be a major player in your life. Also notice the nurses and other staff members within the practice, because they also will be a valuable asset during many of your visits. Be sure to be prepared for your first meeting, and do all that you can to facilitate a good relationship with your ob/gyn.

In order to secure a sound relationship with your physician, be aware of opportunities to keep communication open. Before each visit, write down a list of questions and concerns; between visits, keep a running list of questions—this will improve your chances of getting the most helpful information.

You also should be equipped to take notes on all the suggestions your physician may provide. If you are upset by an event within the office or with any part of your care, be sure to speak with your doctor about it as soon as possible. If you allow the strife to brew, you may lose the good relationship you have worked to achieve.

SAMPLE QUESTIONS
to ask your obsetrician / gynecologist during different stages of your life cycle

* What are my birth control options? Which ones will best protect me against sexually transmitted diseases?

* When should I begin taking prenatal vitamins? Should I take prenatal vitamins while trying to conceive?

* Is this exercise program adequate? What do you recommend to make it more effective?

* Can I continue my workouts during pregnancy?

* How can I best prepare myself physically for childbirth?

* What recommendations do you have concerning the spacing of children?

* What will be the first steps in treating my infertility?

* How aggressively will we try to help me conceive?

* At what age should I stop trying to conceive a child?

* What is a good weight for me at this stage in my life?

* How does my family's health history affect my chances of contracting certain diseases?

A W O M A N ' S R

* What are your suggestions for ideal skin care at my age?

* What screenings/tests will be completed at this appointment, and what will they reveal?

* What are the leading medical problems of women my age? What are the leading causes of death for this same age group?

* When do I need my first mammogram, and how often will I need one?

* What options do I have for approaching menopause in the most effective way?

* Tell me more about the effects of hormone therapy.

* What advice do you have on aging gracefully?

* Do you have the names of other patients who have been faced with this same condition, and who would be willing to share their experience with me?

No question is too personal—this is your opportunity to ask and get answers.

All of the menu plans included in this book are simply suggestions as to what a healthy diet should include. As with any diet, always check with your physician before beginning any weight loss or weight gain strategy.

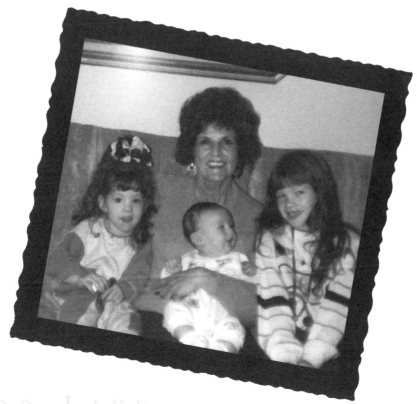

Preconception Care

Schedule a physical with your family doctor, for both you and your partner. Take care of all medical needs, no matter how large or small.

Make an appointment with your dentist, and be sure to take care of x-rays, surgery, or any other procedures.

Plan an appointment with your ob/gyn. Pay close attention to treatment plans for any existing condition. At the examination, be prepared with a list of your own concerns. You should ask some of these questions:

1. What type of birth control should we practice just before we begin trying to conceive?

2. Find out when you may begin taking prenatal vitamins.

3. Find out how to follow your cycle, what your need to document, and how to tell when you are ovulating.

4. Check to see if you are a candidate for genetic screening.

In addition, make sure all of your immunizations are updated.

Both you and your partner should enjoy a healthy diet that is high fiber/low fat/low cholesterol. If you are interested in losing weight, check with your ob/gyn. (Do not go on a crash diet for quick weight loss!)

Continue a regular program of exercise. Be careful not to overexert yourself; this could interfere with ovulation. A scheduled walking program, cycling, or swimming are all good choices. Check with your physician to insure that you have chosen a program compatible with your health needs and your desire to conceive.

Eliminate caffeine, smoking, alcohol, and any illicit drugs. All may greatly decrease your chances of conception. Your partner should also decrease his use, to insure that he can help you to conceive a healthy baby.

Consider the following tests:

* Syphilis	* Hemoglobin or Hematocrit (anemia)
* Gonorrhea	* Rh factor
* Chlamydia	* Urine for sugar or protein
* Herpes	* TB skin test
* HIV	* Hepatitis B

Most importantly, RELAX. Being stressed out or obsessed with getting pregnant may prevent conception altogether.

Morning Sickness Menus Helpers

The following 3 days' worth of menus help to incorporate late evening, high protein snacks, which may help to take the edge off of morning sickness.

Day 1

BREAKFAST
1 bagel or English muffin
1/2 cantaloupe
1 cup skim milk

SNACK
1/2 grapefruit
3 graham cracker squares

LUNCH
1 turkey sandwich:
  2 slices whole wheat bread
  2 slices turkey
  1 slice cheese
  lettuce/tomato/ mustard
1 peach

SNACK
3/4 cup unsweetened cereal
1 cup skim milk

DINNER
1 Georgia Baked Chicken Breast*
1/2 cup wild rice
Honey Baby Carrots*
1 salad with low fat dressing*

HIGH-PROTEIN SNACK
1 cup yogurt
3/4 cup berries

EXTRA SNACK
1 apple

Day 2

BREAKFAST	3/4 cup unsweetened cereal
	1 cup skim milk
	1 cup peaches
SNACK	1 cup yogurt with fruit of your choice
LUNCH	1 cup low fat cottage cheese
	1/2 cantaloupe
	20 seedless grapes
	1 bagel
SNACK	3 graham cracker squares
	1 cup orange juice
DINNER	1/2 cup spaghetti sauce with meat or meatless with
	1/2 cup cheese on top
	1 cup pasta
	1 salad, with low fat dressing*
	1 whole wheat roll
HIGH-PROTEIN SNACK	1 flour tortilla
	1/2 cup refried beans
	2 Tablespoons lite sharp cheddar cheese
EXTRA SNACK	1/2 grapefruit

The ornament of a house is the friends who frequent it.

– Ralph Waldo Emerson

DAY 3

BREAKFAST
1 bagel or English muffin
all-fruit jam
1/2 grapefruit
1 cup skim milk

SNACK
3 graham cracker squares
1 cup orange juice

LUNCH
Greek Salad:
10 to 12 leaves of green leaf lettuce
tomatoes and onions
1/2 cup feta cheese, crumbled
2 Tablespoons light Italian dressing

SNACK
1 cup yogurt
1 cup peaches

DINNER
6 ounce Grilled Seafood Steak*
1 baked potato
spinach, cooked or in a salad
1 cup ice milk

HIGH-PROTEIN SNACK
1 tuna sandwich:
2 slices whole wheat
1/2 cup tuna salad*

EXTRA SNACK
1 apple

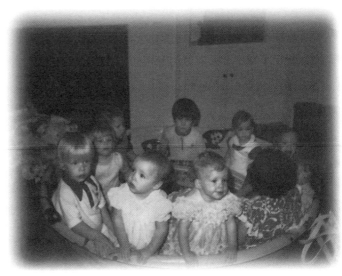

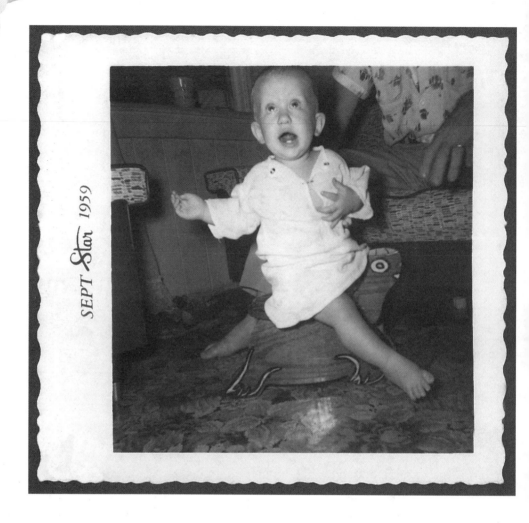

SEPT *Star* 1959

Prenatal Menu Plans

I am not afraid of storms for I am learning to sail my ship.

— Louisa May Alcott

+ Denotes foods that are rich in protein, calcium, iron, or folic acid (all are important for the developing fetus).
* Denotes recipes that are included in this book.

Day 1

BREAKFAST

1 cup unsweetened cereal
1 cup skim milk+
1 banana
1 slice whole wheat toast+
   with all-fruit jam

SNACK	1 peach 3 graham cracker squares

LUNCH	Club sandwich:
	    2 slices whole wheat bread+
	    1 slice low fat or fat free turkey+
	    1 slice 98% fat free ham+
	    1 slice Swiss cheese+
	    lettuce/tomato/mustard
	1/3 cantaloupe+
	2 small oatmeal cookies
	1 cup calcium-added orange juice

SNACK	1/2 cup low fat dressing* for dipping vegetables for dipping
DINNER	4 to 6 Jumbo Stuffed Baked Shells*+ 1/2 cup green beans 1 salad with low fat dressing* 2 rolls
SNACK	1 cup frozen low fat yogurt+ 3/4 cup berries 1 slice angel food cake

DAY 2

BREAKFAST	Egg muffin:
	1 English muffin
	1 egg, scrambled+
	    (use non-stick spray)
	1/4 cup shredded lite sharp
	      cheddar cheese
	1 peach
	1 cup skim milk+

SNACK	1 banana

LUNCH	Chef's salad:
	    2 cups lettuce /tomato /cucumber/
	      carrot mixture+
	    1 slice low fat or fat free turkey+, chopped
	    1 slice 98% fat free ham+, sliced

1 slice Swiss cheese+
1/4 cup shredded lite sharp
cheddar cheese+
12 whole wheat crackers
1/3 cantaloupe+

SNACK   6 graham cracker squares

DINNER   1 Chicken Roll-up*+
1 cup wild rice+
1 cup steamed broccoli+
1 roll

SNACK   1 cup frozen low fat yogurt+

Day 3

BREAKFAST   2 multigrain waffles+ sprinkled with
1 Tablespoon confectioner's sugar
3/4 cup berries
1 cup skim milk+

SNACK   1 cup low fat yogurt+

LUNCH   1 English muffin, halved, top each
half with:
2 Tablespoons pizza sauce
4 Tablespoons mozzarella cheese
2 ounces Canadian bacon rounds or
1 slice 98% fat free ham (Bake at
425 degrees until cheese melts.)
1 tossed salad with low fat dressing*
1 cup calcium-added orange juice+

SNACK   1/3 cantaloupe+

DINNER   1 breast Belle's Best Chicken*+
(save 1 for the next day's lunch)
1 Twice Baked Potato*
1/2 cup green peas+
1/2 cup honey baby carrots*
1 roll

SNACK	1 slice angel food cake
	1 cup low fat frozen yogurt
	1 peach

Day 4

BREAKFAST	1 cup unsweetened cereal
	1 cup skim milk+
	1 banana
	1 slice whole wheat toast+ with
	all-fruit jam

| SNACK | 1 cup low fat yogurt+ |
| | 1 peach |

LUNCH	Mexican Salad:
	2 cups lettuce+
	1 tomato, diced
	1 chicken breast+, cut into chunks
	(chicken from night before)
	1/2 cup shredded lite sharp
	cheddar cheese+
	2 Tablespoon lite sour cream
	Southland Salsa*
	16 baked tortilla chips

| SNACK | 1 cup pretzels |

DINNER	2 cups Low Fat Macaroni and
	Cheese*+
	1/2 cup green beans+
	1/2 cup summer squash
	1 sliced tomato

| SNACK | 1 frozen fruit bar |

Day 5

BREAKFAST

Egg muffin:
1 English muffin
1 egg + , scrambled in non-stick
    spray
1/4 cup shredded lite sharp
        cheddar cheese+
1 apple
1 cup skim milk +

SNACK

1 cup melon cubes

LUNCH

turkey sandwich:
2 slices whole wheat bread +
2 slices low fat or fat free turkey +
lettuce/tomato/mustard
1 banana
1 cup calcium-added orange juice

SNACK

1 bagel with
1 Tablespoon low fat cream cheese

DINNER

1 breast+, marinated and grilled in
    fat free Italian dressing
    (save one for tomorrow's lunch)
1 cup Marinated Broccoli Salad*+
1 cup baked zucchini wedges
1 cob of corn

SNACK

1 cup low fat frozen yogurt +
1 slice angel food cake

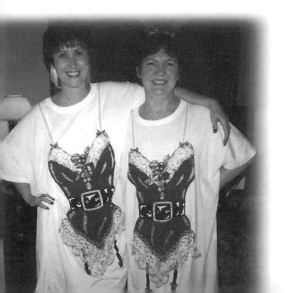

Day 6

BREAKFAST	1 cup unsweetened cereal
	1 cup skim milk +
	1 banana
	1 slice whole wheat toast + , with all-fruit jam
SNACK	1 bagel with
	1 Tablespoon low fat cream cheese
LUNCH	1 grilled chicken salad:
	2 cups lettuce /tomato /cucumber/ carrot mixture +
	1 breast Italian grilled chicken + , from night before
	1/4 cup shredded lite sharp cheddar cheese
	Honey Mustard Dressing
	1 cup calcium-added orange juice
SNACK	1/2 cup low fat dressing*
	1 cup pretzels
DINNER	2 cups Chicken Pot Pie* +
	1 sliced tomato
	1 cup pineapple chunks
	1 roll
SNACK	1 cup low fat frozen yogurt +
	3/4 cup berries

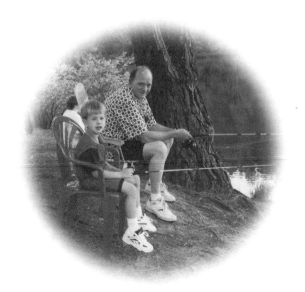

Whoever is happy will make others happy too.

– Anne Frank

Day 7

BREAKFAST

2 multigrain waffles + , sprinkled with
1 Tablespoon confectioner's sugar
3/4 cup berries
1 cup skim milk+

SNACK

1 cup apple sauce, no sugar added
6 graham cracker squares

LUNCH

Ham sandwich:
2 slices whole wheat bread +
2 slices 98% fat free ham +
1 slice Swiss cheese +
lettuce/tomato/mustard
1 cup apple sauce
2 oatmeal cookies

SNACK

1/2 cup low fat dressing*
    for dipping
vegetables+ for dipping

DINNER

2 Salmon Croquettes* +
1/2 cup cheese grits*
1 cup cole slaw*
1 tomato, sliced

SNACK

1 cup low fat frozen
    yogurt +
1 slice angel food cake
1 peach

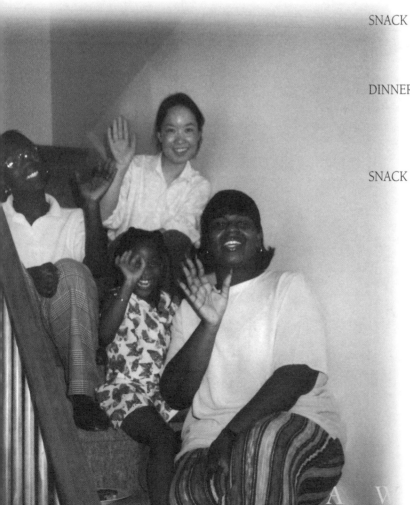

Miscarriage

For many reasons, miscarriage can be a very lonely time for a woman. One depressing reality is that much of our society does not view miscarriage as an actual death of a "real" person. Even though the baby did not live, a woman becomes a mother as soon as she knows she is pregnant. We begin to make plans about how we will tell everyone, whether "it" is a girl or a boy, what names we like, where to put the nursery, and the list goes on and on. The baby is very real to the parents, and especially to the mother, who is growing life inside of her. When that life is lost, part of her dies.

Fathers, too, grieve over the loss; many times in very different ways than the mother, so it is imperative to be sensitive to each other, and give each other ample time to grieve.

Although the mother's grief may be more intense, the key to healing comes with open communication on the part of both parents.

Many women worry that they did something wrong that caused the miscarriage; that somehow the loss was their fault. This is a very normal reaction. The fact is that most miscarriages occur very early in pregnancy, and are the body's reaction to a embryo that is developing abnormally. Even though this is reality, it does not provide much comfort.

The apprehension a woman endures during the next pregnancy is yet another component in her journey of grief. She may be afraid to get too excited about the growing fetus in order to protect herself from the overwhelming heartache of the previous miscarriage. One helpful suggestion is to set small goals to work toward during the pregnancy; as each is realized, she can concentrate on the next one.

Although the loss of a baby will always be felt by the mother, time seems to be the key in healing the emotional injury. Another source of comfort is the support of others who have experienced the same type of loss. A support group such as The Compassionate Friends, Inc. can provide information, group meetings, and possibly phone support.

If you have a friend or relative who has had a miscarriage, here are some things NOT to say:

"It will be for the best."

"God needed another little angel, so He took your baby."

"Something good will come out of this."

"At least you already have a child; think of those without children."

"It wasn't really a baby."

"Try your best not to think about it, pretend it didn't happen."

"I know just how you feel."

The most supportive thing you can do is to give a hug, or just say:

"I am so sorry."

"This must be the worse thing you've ever experienced."

"I am here if you want to talk."

"I am praying for you."

"I am thinking of you."

A small gesture of kindness also will be appreciated. Don't ask if there is anything you can do, just do it. Bring over a meal to the family, send a plant or small tree in memory of the baby, clean her house so she can rest, offer to make any needed phone calls or errands, listen when she wants to talk, and allow her to grieve according to her own timetable.

The following books will offer additional comfort:

Allen, Marie. *Miscarriage: Women Sharing From The Heart.* John Wiley and Sons, 1993.

Berezin, Nancy. *After A Loss In Pregnancy.* Simon and Schuster, 1982.

Borg, Susan and Lasker, Judith. *When Pregnancy Fails.* Beacon Press, 1981.

Friedman, Rochelle, and Gradstein, Bonnie. *Surviving Pregnancy Loss.* Little Brown and Company, 1982.

Schwiert, Pat and Kirk, Paul. *When Hello Means Goodbye.* University of Oregon Health Sciences Center, 1981.

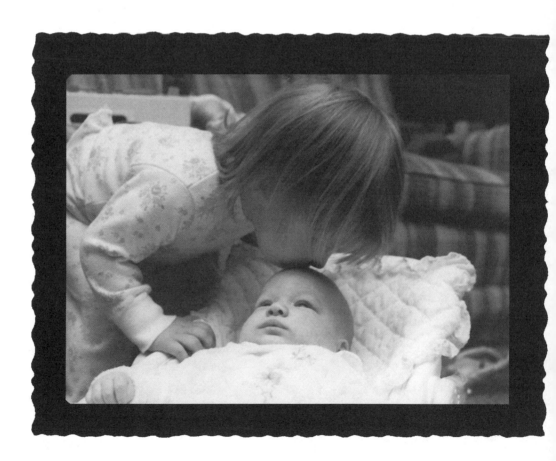

Infertility

One of the most desperate feelings for a couple must be the realization that the hope of pregnancy is not going as planned. We live in a society where we meticulously design the biggest events of our lives. We are advised to make clear, precise education choices; we become engaged and plan a wedding; we set goals and map out plans; we create homes, and we have dreams. Unfortunately, for some couples, the dream of parenthood is thwarted by the possibility of infertility.

Infertility is defined as the inability of a couple to conceive after more than one year of unprotected sex, or the inability to deliver a live baby. Facing infertility will be the most challenging aspect of a couple's life, both physically and emotionally.

The following suggestions may prove helpful if you suspect that you are having difficulty conceiving:

Make an appointment with your gynecologist if you have been practicing unprotected sex for more than one year, and you have not conceived. If you are over thirty, you may seek the advice of a physician after only six months of unprotected sex and no conception.

Keep an accurate diary of your cycle, as well as times and dates of intercourse; this may be helpful information for your physician.

In addition to a physical exam, you will most likely endure lab work, as well as diagnostic studies. At times, you may feel like you no longer own your body or your sexual relationship. This is a very natural feeling.

Investigate your health insurance plan to see what part of infertility testing and treatments will be covered. You will want to know what is covered by your plan before your first doctor's appointment.

Make sure you get all of the facts. Keep a notebook with you to jot down questions that concern you or your partner.

Be a good listener; and consider all options. Try to accomplish open communication with your mate so that any decision will be based on how the two of you feel.

Find a support group. Ask your physician's office, call a community help line, or inquire at your local hospital to find such a support group. If there is none in your area, ask your physician if she would help you reach another infertility patient.

Form a good response to the question, "When are your going to start a family?"

Maintain other parts of your life; try not to let the infertility engulf you and your husband.

SUGGESTED READINGS:

Rosenberg, Helane and Epstein, Yakov. *Getting Pregnant When You Thought You Couldn't.* Warner Books, 1993.

Shulgold, Barbara and Sipiora, Lynne. *In Search of Motherhood.* Dell Publishing, 1995.

Silber, Sherman. *How To Get Pregnant With the New Technology.* Warner Books, 1991.

Tan, S.L.; Jacobs, Howard; and Seibel, Machelle. *Infertility: Your Questions Answered.* Carol Publishing, 1995.

Adoption

Adoption is the answer to many couples' quest to begin a family. There are a variety of reasons for choosing adoption, and fortunately, these adoptive parents are available to provide nurturing homes to children who otherwise may live in less fortunate circumstances.

If you are considering adoption, you need to consider the following:

* Are you prepared to make a lifetime commitment to a child?
* Will you provide unconditional love?
* How young a child would you like to adopt?
* Would you consider international adoption?

When you have answered these questions, and you feel that adoption is right for your family, you need to design a plan that includes:

How you will let everyone know that you are wanting to adopt. This includes putting your name on as many adoption lists as possible.

Seeking an attorney who is trained in adoption or family law.

Taking a parenting class.

Obtaining information on the costs that will be involved, and then budgeting so that you are prepared.

Exploring support systems such as a support group, a counselor, your church family, or someone who has been touched by adoption.

The accompanying book list can help you find many answers on your own, as well as detailing information about what you may need to do in order to make adoption a reality.

Alexander-Roberts, Colleen. *The Essential Adoption Handbook.* 1993.

Beauvais-Godwin and Godwin, Raymond. *The Independent Adoption Manual: From Beginning to Baby.* 1993.

Crain, Connie and Duffy, Janice. *How To Adopt a Child: A Comprehensive Guide For Prospective Parents.* 1994.

Gilman, Lois. *The Adoption Resource Book.* 1992.

Hicks, Randall. *Adopting in America: How to Adopt Within One Year.* 1993.

Martin, Cynthia. *Beating the Adoption Game.* 1988.

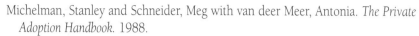

Michelman, Stanley and Schneider, Meg with van deer Meer, Antonia. *The Private Adoption Handbook.* 1988.

Sifferman, Kelly Allen. *Adoption: A Legal Guide For Birth and Adoptive Parents.* 1994.

Takas, Marianne and Warner, Edward. *To Love a Child.* 1992.

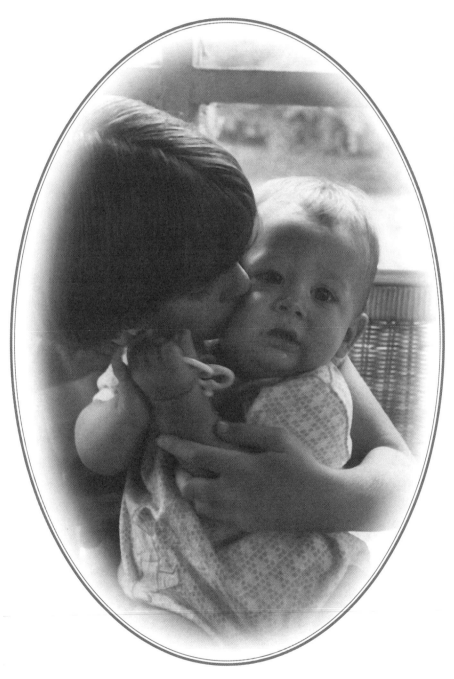

Love just doesn't sit there, like a stone, it has to be made, like bread; re-made all the time, made new.

– Ursula K. Le Guin

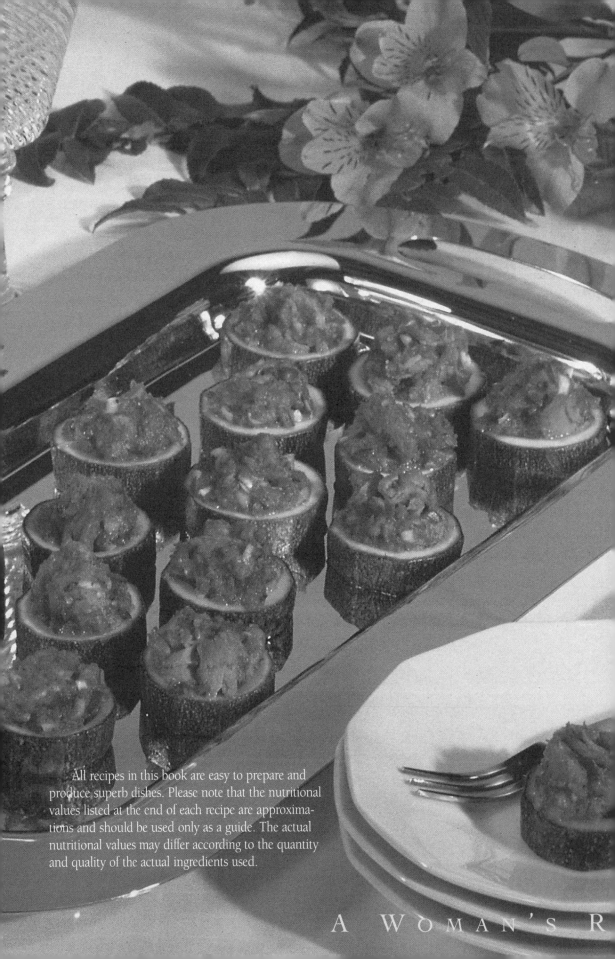

All recipes in this book are easy to prepare and produce superb dishes. Please note that the nutritional values listed at the end of each recipe are approximations and should be used only as a guide. The actual nutritional values may differ according to the quantity and quality of the actual ingredients used.

LOW FAT CELEBRATION CHEESE BALL

2 8-ounce packages fat-free cream cheese, softened
1 can crushed pineapple
1/2 cup pecan chips
1 green pepper, finely diced
2 teaspoons seasoned salt
2 cups crushed pretzels

  Combine softened cream cheese, drained pineapple, pecan chips, green
  pepper, and seasoned salt. Mix well.
  Form into a ball; roll in crushed pretzels.
  Refrigerate for at least 24 hours; may be frozen and thawed before serving.
  Serve with low fat or fat-free crackers.
Yields: 10 1/2-cup servings; calories: 188; total fat: 5g; saturated fat: 1g; choles-
terol: 3mg; sodium: 1036mg; carbohydrates: 27g; calcium: 151mg; iron; 1mg.

MEXICAN PARTY DIP

4 cups Vegetarian Chili*
1 block reduced fat Velveeta cheese
   baked tortilla chips

  Place chili in a crock pot, turn on high.
  Slice Velveeta into cubes.
  Add cubes to chili, stir frequently until cheese melts.
  Serve hot with chips for dipping.
Yields: 10 1/2-cup servings; calories: 166; total fat: 8g; saturated fat: 1g; choles-
terol: 10mg; sodium: 734mg; carbohydrates: 10g; calcium: 192mg; iron: 1mg.

HOT CRAB DIP

8 ounces low fat cream cheese
1 can white crab meat

1 teaspoon horseradish
2 green onions, chopped
2 Tablespoons skim milk
1 teaspoon salt
1/2 cup Parmesan cheese
buttery flavored non-stick spray

Combine cream cheese, crab, horseradish, onions, skim milk, and salt.
Mix well and pour into casserole coated with buttery spray.
Sprinkle with Parmesan cheese and spray with buttery spray.
Bake at 350 degrees for 30 minutes.
Yields: 8 2-ounce servings; calories: 100; total fat: 7g; saturated fat: 4g; cholesterol: 23mg; sodium: 483mg; carbohydrates: 3g; calcium: 128mg; iron: 1mg.

CUCUMBER DILL DIP

1 16-ounce container lite sour cream
1 cucumber, unpeeled, scrubbed, and diced
2 teaspoons dill weed
1/2 teaspoon salt

Combine all ingredients, blend well.
Serve with raw vegetables for dipping.
Yields: 8 1/2-cup servings; calories: 79; total fat: 5g; saturated fat: 4g; cholesterol: 18mg; sodium: 171mg; carbohydrates: 5g; calcium: 83mg; iron: 0mg.

SPINACH QUESADILLAS

4 large flour tortillas
1 box frozen spinach, thawed and drained
1 red onion, chopped
4 Tablespoons sliced jalapeno peppers (optional)
2 cups shredded low fat Monterey Jack cheese
  Southland Salsa*

Place 1/4 of the spinach, 1/4 of the onion, 1 Tablespoon jalapeno peppers, and 1 cup of cheese on one half of each jumbo tortilla.
Fold tortilla in half.
Bake at 350 degrees for 20 to 30 minutes.
Serve with salsa on top.
Yields: 4 servings; calories: 434; total fat: 22g; saturated fat: 14g; cholesterol: 81mg; sodium: 1158mg; carbohydrates: 20g; calcium: 1110mg; iron: 2mg.

MINI CHICKEN-FILLED POCKETS

6 chicken breasts, boiled and boned
1 large Vidalia onion, grated
1 8-ounce package light cream cheese, softened
1 Tablespoon reduced-fat margarine
1 teaspoon salt
1 teaspoon pepper
1 tube refrigerated crescent rolls
   buttery flavored non-stick spray
   fresh parsley

   Tear chicken into very small, bite-sized pieces.
   Combine chicken, onion, cream cheese, margarine, salt, and pepper;
   mix well.
   Unroll crescent dough, and divide the 8 pre-cut triangles.
   Cut each triangle in half, and press until very thin.
   Place a scoop of chicken mixture onto each thin dough piece.
   Wrap the dough neatly around the chicken mixture.
   Spray the top of each packet with buttery flavored non-stick spray.
   Bake at 350 for 30 minutes, or until browned.
   Garnish with parsley sprig.
Yields: 16 servings; calories: 116; total fat; 4g; saturated fat: 1g; cholesterol: 33mg;
sodium: 391mg; carbohydrates: 8g; calcium: 19mg; iron: 1mg.

CHEESE WAFERS

2 sticks regular margarine, softened
2 cups shredded sharp cheddar cheese
2 cups all-purpose flour
1/4 teaspoon cayenne pepper
2 cups Rice Krispies

   Cream together margarine and cheese.
   Add flour, cayenne pepper, and Rice Krispies.
   Mix until well blended.
   Roll into small balls, then pat into small round wafers.
   Bake at 425 degrees for 20 minutes.
Yields: 25 servings; calories: 141; total fat: 10g; saturated fat: 3g; cholesterol: 10g;
sodium: 131mg; carbohydrates: 10g; calcium: 67mg; iron: 1mg.

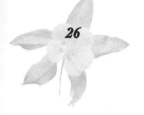

DRINKS

APPLE PUNCH

1 64-ounce bottle apple juice
1 2-liter bottle ginger ale
strawberries
    Chill apple juice and ginger ale; combine just before serving.
    Garnish with fresh strawberries.
Yields: 20 1-cup servings; calories: 84; total fat: 0g; saturated fat: 0g; cholesterol:
0mg; sodium: 10mg; carbohydrates: 21g; calcium: 11mg; iron: 1mg.

PEPPERMINT HOT COCOA

1 package hot cocoa mix
1 mug water
1 peppermint stick
    Combine cocoa mix and hot water.
    Stir with peppermint stick until stick is melted.
Yields: 1 1-cup serving; calories: 132; total fat: 1g; saturated fat: 1g; cholesterol: 1
mg; sodium: 150mg; carbohydrates: 22g; calcium: 97mg; iron: 0mg.

REFRESHING FRUIT PUNCH

1 quart orange juice
1 quart pineapple juice
1 quart lemonade
1 quart limeade
6 liters Sprite
fresh fruit
    Combine all ingredients.
    Serve in punch bowl garnished with fresh fruit.
Yields: 44 1-cup servings; calories: 93; total fat: 0g; saturated fat: 0g; cholesterol:
0mg; sodium: 19mg; carbohydrates: 24g; calcium: 9mg; iron: 0mg.

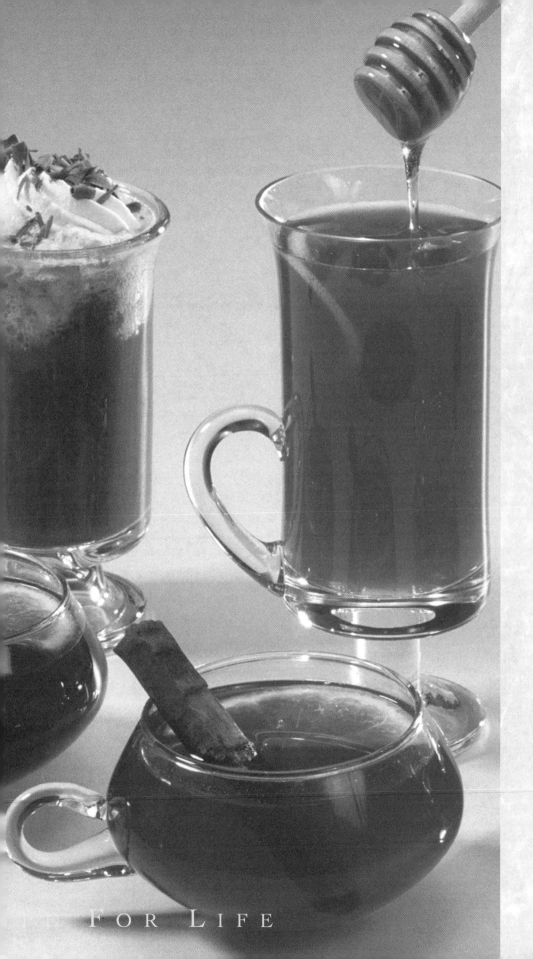

DRINKS

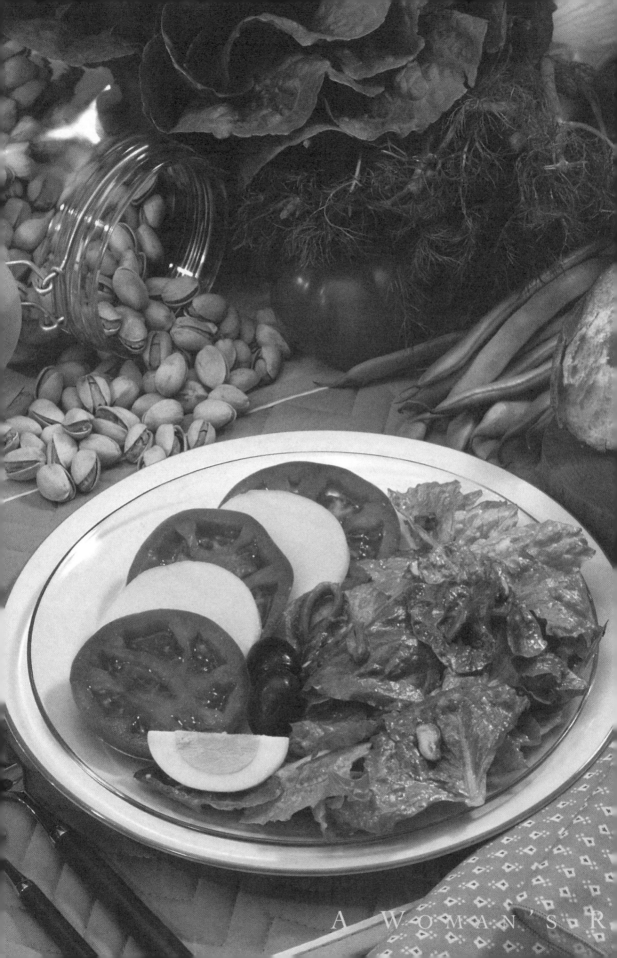

CHICKEN ALMOND SALAD

4 skinless chicken breasts, boiled, boned, and diced
1 small can crushed pineapple, do not drain
1/2 cup low cholesterol mayonnaise
1/2 cup toasted almonds
1 teaspoon salt
1 teaspoon black pepper

Combine all ingredients.
Add a touch more mayonnaise, salt, and pepper, if necessary.

Yields: 8 1/2-cup servings. Per serving: calories: 308; total fat: 12g; saturated fat: 2g; cholesterol: 40mg; sodium: 374mg; carbohydrates: 10g; calcium: 52mg; iron: 1mg.

MEXICAN LAYERED SALAD

3 cups cooked, diced chicken breasts
1 package taco seasoning mix
2 cans fat-free refried beans
1 cup low cholesterol mayonnaise
1 cup lite sour cream
3 cups shredded lettuce
2 large, fresh tomatoes, diced
2 cups shredded, lite sharp cheddar cheese
salsa, optional
baked tortilla chips

Place layer of chicken in 9 x 13 casserole dish.
Sprinkle chicken with 1/2 of the taco seasoning mix.
Add layer of refried beans.
Combine mayonnaise, sour cream, and remaining taco seasoning mix.
Layer sour cream mixture over beans.
Complete layering with lettuce, tomato, and cheese on top.
Serve with baked tortilla chips and salsa.

Yields: 10 1-cup servings; calories: 381, total fat: 17g, saturated fat: 8g, cholesterol: 95mg, sodium: 805mg, carbohydrates: 18g, calcium: 383mg, iron: 2mg.

GUACAMOLE SALAD

2 ripe avocados
1 lemon
2 Tablespoons low cholesterol mayonnaise
1 teaspoon garlic powder
1 teaspoon chili powder

Slice avocados lengthwise.
Remove pit, and scoop out avocado with a spoon.
Immediately sprinkle avocado with the juice from the lemon.
Mash the avocado with a potato masher or fork.
Add the other ingredients.
Mix well. Serve on a bed of lettuce, or as a dip.

Yields: 8 1/4-cup servings. Per serving: calories: 94; total fat: 9g; saturated fat: 1g; cholesterol: 1mg; sodium: 28mg; carbohydrates: 5g; calcium: 9mg; iron: .62mg.

SHRIMP SALAD

1 pound medium shrimp, boiled and peeled
1/2 cup low cholesterol mayonnaise
1 Tablespoon horseradish
1 stalk celery, diced
6-8 cherry tomatoes, quartered
1 lemon, halved
1 teaspoon salt

Combine shrimp, mayonnaise, horseradish, celery, and tomatoes.
Add juice from 1/2 of the lemon, and the salt.
Toss until well coated.
Serve on lettuce, or if shrimp is diced, use as a sandwich filling.
Use remaining lemon half to make lemon curl garnish.

Yields: 4 3/4-cup servings. Per serving: calories: 259; total fat: 12g; saturated fat: 2g; cholesterol: 215mg; sodium: 1265mg; carbohydrates: 9g; calcium: 82mg; iron: 4mg.

CURRIED TURKEY SALAD

 8 slices fat-free turkey, cut into julienne slices
20 red seedless grapes, halved
 1 very small onion, diced
 2 stalks celery, diced
1/2 cup plain non-fat yogurt
1/2 cup low cholesterol mayonnaise
 3 teaspoons curry powder
 3 Granny Smith apples, cored and chopped into bite-sized pieces*
 2 Tablespoons lemon juice

Combine turkey, grapes, onion, and celery; toss.
Mix yogurt, mayonnaise, and curry powder; blend well.
Add yogurt mixture to turkey mixture; toss to coat evenly.
Peel and chop apples just before serving, and sprinkle with lemon juice.
Add apples to salad and serve on lettuce.
* If you make the salad ahead of time, chop and add apples just before serving.

Yields: 10 1/2-cup servings. Per serving: calories: 88; total fat: 3g; saturated fat: .5g; cholesterol: 11mg; sodium: 315mg; carbohydrates: 12g; calcium: 33mg; iron: .3mg.

ITALIAN CUCUMBER/TOMATO SALAD

 3 fresh cucumbers, scrubbed well
 3 vine ripe tomatoes, washed well
 1 large sweet Vidalia onion, sliced into rings
1/2 cup white vinegar
1/2 cup blush wine
 1 Tablespoon virgin olive oil
 1 Tablespoon sugar
 1 teaspoon oregano
 1 teaspoon crushed basil
1/2 teaspoon salt
 1 teaspoon pepper

Scrape the skin of each cucumber, lengthwise, to form ridges when sliced.
Thinly slice cucumber.
Chop tomatoes into thick chunks.

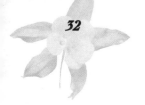

Combine cucumber slices, tomato chunks, and onion rings in a large bowl.
Blend remaining ingredients in a separate bowl.
Pour dressing over salad mixture. Toss until evenly coated.

Yields: 6 1-cup servings. Per serving: calories: 67; total fat: 2g; saturated fat: .3g; cholesterol: 0mg; sodium: 141mg; carbohydrates: 10g; calcium: 30mg; iron: 1mg.

MEXICAN BEAN SALAD

1 cup cooked Spanish rice*
1 cup cooked black beans or 1 can black beans
1 can whole kernel corn, drained
2 tomatoes, diced
1 green peppers, diced
1/2 cup Southern Salsa
1/2 teaspoon garlic powder
1/2 teaspoon chili powder
shredded lite sharp cheddar cheese
lite sour cream

Combine all ingredients, except cheese and sour cream.
Toss until well blended.
Refrigerate at least 1 hour before serving.
Serve on lettuce, garnished with 1 Tablespoon lite sharp cheddar, and
1 Tablespoon lite sour cream.

Yields: 6 3/4-cup servings. Per serving: calories: 145; total fat: 5g; saturated fat: 3g; cholesterol: 15mg; sodium: 291mg; carbohydrates: 18g; calcium: 166mg; iron: 1mg.

MARINATED BROCCOLI SALAD

1 bunch fresh broccoli, washed and flowerettes cut into bite-sized pieces
1/2 cup raisins
3/4 cup low cholesterol mayonnaise
1/3 cup white vinegar
1/4 cup sugar

Toss together broccoli and raisins.
Mix mayonnaise, vinegar, and sugar; blend well.
Pour dressing over broccoli; toss to coat well.
Serve chilled.
For variation, add 2 Tablespoons chopped red onion, or 2 Tablespoons crumbled bacon or Bacos.

Yields: 4 to 5 1/2-cup servings. Per serving: calories: 234; total fat: 9g; saturated fat: 1.6g; cholesterol: 11mg; sodium: 244mg; carbohydrates: 39g; calcium: 26mg; iron: .7mg.

SOUTHERN POTATO SALAD

3 cups cooked and cubed potatoes
2 Tablespoons chopped green onions
2 stalks celery, chopped
1 2-ounce jar diced pimento
1/2 cup plain non-fat yogurt
2 Tablespoons French's Bold & Spicy mustard
1 teaspoon sugar
1 teaspoon white vinegar
1/8 teaspoon garlic powder
1 teaspoon black pepper
   paprika

Combine potatoes, green onion, celery, and pimento in large bowl.
Blend remaining ingredients in a separate bowl.
Pour dressing over potato mixture, toss until well coated.
Sprinkle with paprika. Serve chilled.

Yields: 6 to 7 1/2-cup servings. Per serving: calories: 100; total fat: .4g; saturated fat: 0g; cholesterol: .4mg; sodium: 91mg; carbohydrates: 22g; calcium: 55mg; iron: .7mg.

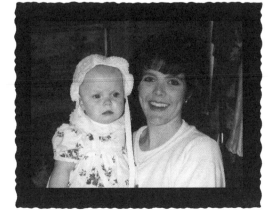

GREEK PASTA SALAD

1 box tri-colored pasta swirls, cooked and drained
1 can pitted black olives, drained
1 cup sliced mushrooms
1/2 cup crumbled feta cheese
1 1/2 cup fat-free Italian dressing

    Combine pasta, black olives, mushrooms, and feta cheese; toss well.
    Blend dressing mix, oil, vinegar, and water.
    Pour dressing over pasta; toss to coat evenly.

Yields: 8 1/2-cup servings. Per serving: calories: 152; total fat: 6g; saturated fat: 2g; cholesterol: 6mg; sodium: 850mg; carbohydrates: 21g; calcium: 46mg; iron: .8mg.

COLE SLAW

1 head of cabbage, shredded
1 onion, diced
1 carrot, shredded
1 cup fat-free plain yogurt
1/2 cup low cholesterol mayonnaise
1/4 cup white wine vinegar
2 Tablespoons sugar
1 teaspoon salt
1 teaspoon pepper
1 teaspoon dill weed

    Combine all ingredients, and toss well to coat.
    Refrigerate overnight.

Yields: 8 3/4-cup servings. Per serving: calories: 89; total fat: .5g; saturated fat: 1g; cholesterol: .6mg; sodium: 479mg; carbohydrates: 18g; calcium: 139mg; iron: 1mg.

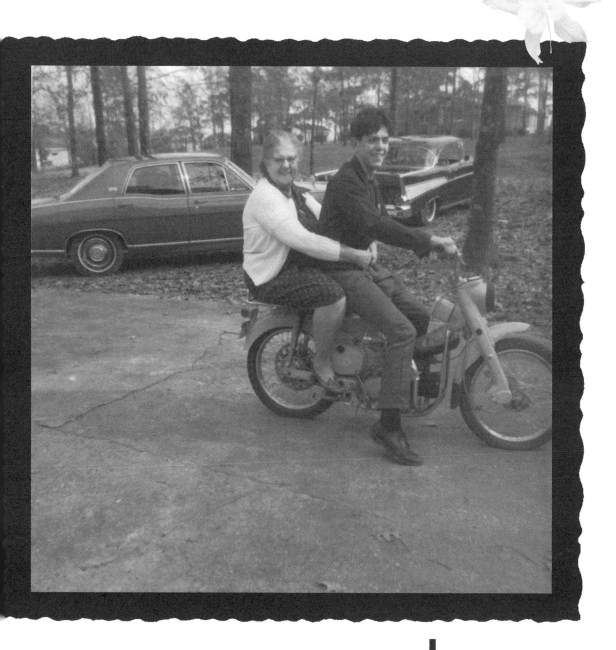

It is not the years
in your life but the
life in your years
that counts!

– *Adlai Stevenson*

36

TERRIFIC TUNA SALAD

1 can water packed tuna, drained
2 Tablespoons low cholesterol mayonnaise
1 Tablespoon dill pickle cubes
1/2 teaspoon tarragon
1/2 teaspoon dill weed
1/4 teaspoon black pepper

Mix all ingredients together.
Store in air-tight container.

Yields: 2 1/2-cup servings. Per serving: calories: 130; total fat: 4g; saturated fat: .7g; cholesterol: 27mg; sodium: 437mg; carbohydrates: 3g; calcium: 28mg; iron: 2mg.

BLEU CHEESE DRESSING

1 cup plain non-fat yogurt
2 Tablespoons lite sour cream
4 ounces bleu cheese chunks, crumbled
1 teaspoon Worcestershire sauce
dash hot sauce
1 teaspoon garlic powder or garlic salt

Combine all ingredients, blend well.
Add just enough skim milk if necessary for desired consistency.

Yields: 20 2-Tablespoon servings. Per serving: calories: 42; total fat: 3g; saturated fat: 2g; cholesterol: 7mg; sodium: 132mg; carbohydrates: 2g; calcium: 81mg; iron: 0mg.

FETA CHEESE VINAIGRETTE

1 packet Italian dressing mix
3/4 cup olive or canola oil
1/3 cup white vinegar

1/4 cup water
3/4 cup crumbled feta cheese

    Combine all ingredients in air-tight jar.
    Shake well.

Yields: 25 2-Tablespoon servings. Per serving: calories: 88; total fat: 8g; saturated fat: 2g; cholesterol: 6mg; sodium: 190mg: carbohydrates: 3g; calcium: 37mg; iron: 0mg.

LOW FAT RANCH

1 package ranch-style dressing mix
1 cup plain non-fat yogurt
1/2 cup skim milk
1/2 cup low cholesterol mayonnaise

    Combine all ingredients.
    Blend well. Refrigerate for 1 or more hours before serving.

Yields: 26 2-Tablespoon servings. Per serving: calories: 22; total fat: 0g; saturated fat: 0g; cholesterol: .3mg; sodium: 130mg; carbohydrates: 4g; calcium: 25mg; iron: 0mg.

CREAMY HERB DRESSING

2 cups plain non-fat yogurt
1 teaspoon crushed basil
1 teaspoon crushed rosemary
1/2 teaspoon dill weed
pinch of sugar

    Combine all ingredients.
    Blend well.

Yields: 17 2-Tablespoon servings. Per serving: calories: 18; total fat: 0g; saturated fat: 0g; cholesterol: .5mg; sodium: 22mg; carbohydrates: 3g; calcium: 61mg; iron: .1mg.

CINNAMON FRUIT DRESSING

1 cup fat-free or lite sour cream
1 Tablespoon cinnamon
2 teaspoons sugar

Blend all ingredients together.
Serve as a topping for fruit or as a dip.

Yields: 9 2-Tablespoon servings. Per serving: calories: 41; total fat: 2g; saturated fat: 2g; cholesterol: 9mg; sodium: 18mg; carbohydrates: 3g; calcium: 45mg; iron: .3mg.

HONEY MUSTARD DRESSING

1 cup honey
1 cup French's Bold & Spicy mustard

Combine and blend until smooth.
(Great on grilled chicken or baked potatoes.)

Yields: 20 2-Tablespoon servings. Per serving: calories: 61; total fat: .6g; saturated fat 0g; cholesterol: 0mg; sodium: 157mg; carbohydrates: 15g; calcium: 12mg; iron: 0mg.

LOW FAT 1000 ISLAND DRESSING

1/2 cup plain non-fat yogurt
1/2 cup low cholesterol mayonnaise
1/2 cup ketchup
 2 Tablespoons dill pickle cubes
1/2 teaspoon garlic salt
1/2 teaspoon pepper
dash of hot sauce

Combine all ingredients, blend well.
Chill before serving.

Yields: 14 2-Tablespoon servings. Per serving: calories: 23; total fat: 0g; saturated fat: 0g; cholesterol: .1mg; sodium: 207mg; carbohydrates: 5g; calcium: 22mg; iron: .1mg.

CUCUMBER SAUCE

1 large cucumber, finely diced
2 cups fat-free or lite sour cream
1 packet ranch-style dressing mix

    Combine all ingredients, blend well.
    Serve with grilled seafood, raw vegetables, or as a dressing.

Yields: 45 2-Tablespoon servings. Per serving: calories: 28; total fat: 1g; saturated fat: 1g; cholesterol: 4mg; sodium: 103mg; carbohydrates: 4g; calcium: 15mg; iron: 0mg.

SOUTHLAND SALSA

1 large can crushed tomatoes or 2 - 3 vine-ripe tomatoes, crushed
1 large Vidalia onion, finely diced
1 green pepper, finely diced
1 small can diced mild green chili peppers
4 jalapeno peppers, diced (optional)
2 teaspoons garlic salt
   hot sauce to taste
    Combine all ingredients and chill.

Yields: 20 2-Tablespoon servings. Per serving: calories: 8; total fat: 0g; saturated fat: 0g; cholesterol: 0mg; sodium: 102mg; carbohydrates: 2g; calcium: 6mg; iron: 0mg.

The
Meat
Of
The

Age sits with decent grace upon his visage, And worthily becomes his silver locks; He bears the marks of many years well spent, Of virtue truth well tried, and wise experience.

– Rowe.

Matter

IPE FOR LIFE

Negotiating A Parental Leave

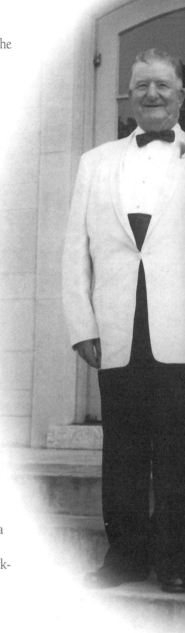

A s the number of dual career families increases, the balance between work and family becomes an ongoing issue. One of the first times a couple will be faced with family policy in the workplace is during the planning for a parental leave for the birth of a child.

In the past, many women felt fortunate to have jobs, therefore, they took whatever leave plan was given to them. Today, women are a vital part of many companies, so they have more room for negotiation when considering a maternity leave.

Questions to ask Yourself Before Planning Your Leave

Do you enjoy your job, and how much is your job a part of you?

Are you interested in other jobs/positions or do you wish to stay on the same career path?

Is your position essential to your company, and are you essential to that position?

What is the standard maternity leave for others in the same or similar positions?

Will you receive employee benefits during an unpaid leave?

Would you consider returning to work on a part-time basis?

Does your employer offer flextime or a work-share program?

Throughout the process of negotiating, planning, enjoying, and returning to work from your leave, always keep a professional attitude at work. The more proficient you are on the job, the better your chances of negotiating a good leave. Determine how long your family can survive without your income, make sure you are familiar with the benefits offered to parents today. Also, investigate what options may be available to you.

Find a trustworthy friend with whom to discuss some of your ideas with before you present them to your employer. Work out a good leave plan with yourself first, then present the leave plan to your partner; after you both have decided on what is best for your family, arrange a meeting with your boss and negotiate the best leave possible.

If you are going to propose a truly novel plan, you also may want to propose a trial period for a few days, in which you will work the new schedule. During the trial run, keep accurate records of your accomplishments and then report back to your employer. A novel plan that works will open the door to others in the future.

Some different options to consider:

Returning part-time at first, then gradually adding more time. For example, return 2 days a week at 6 weeks, increase to 3 days at 8 weeks, 4 days at 10 weeks, and a full 5-day week at 12 weeks.

Return five days a week, but for fewer hours daily.

Work half-time at the office, half-time at home.

Begin working 20 hours a week at 12 weeks, 30 hours a week at 18 weeks, and then a 40-hour week at 24 weeks.

See if there is someone who may want to share your job with you. A good work-share program can be beneficial to all involved.

Be prepared when you meet with your employer.

I am part of all that I have met.

– Alfred, Lord Tennyson

When presenting your plan for your parental leave, emphasize how valuable you are to the company. Be sure to be a good listener; your employer may have some ideas that you have not even considered. Wait at least a day before you make the final decision, and be sure you have considered all the aspects of your leave.

When negotiating your leave, ask for more than you expect to get in order to have some bargaining room. Find out what others at the same level have received, and seek the same leave, or have another idea that is so good, it probably will be given a chance.

Be sure to consider your employer's point of view. Be sure to take all the leave to which you are entitled; you may be able to add vacation days or sick days if they are available to you. Check with your employer about the policy concerning which days must be used first.

If you will be receiving a paid leave, find out when your checks will be mailed. Will it be on the same schedule as your regular paychecks?

Be careful how much at-home work you agree to do while on your leave. You may find out that you don't have as much time as you thought. Remember, you can always request more work once you see how much you can handle.

If you are going to suggest bringing the baby to work, be sure you have a job that will complement that decision, as well as the space at work to accommodate the baby and baby's equipment. You also must set the date when you will stop bringing the baby to work. This can be a workable situation, but you definitely will need your employer's support.

While meeting with your employer, determine when your last day of work will occur, and find out what is expected to be completed before your leave begins. Make sure you understand every part of your leave plan. Be sure to put your agreement in writing.

Before you begin your leave, find a confidante at work upon whom you can rely to keep you posted on office happenings. This person also will be helpful during your transition back to work.

Be sure to document all of your preparations for your leave, and keep a file; this way you will have a record of all of your actions. Make sure your co-workers know that you are planning to return to work. Find out how you can ease your co-workers' adjustment to your absence, and assure them that you are still part of the team.

Save your last week to tie up any loose ends. Be sure to leave your work organized each day, so that someone else could step in if the baby comes early.

Make child care arrangements long before your leave begins. Do some reading on infant and child development so that you will know what to expect from a high-quality child care provider. Be sure to establish a good relationship with your baby's caregiver.

In addition to securing child care, select a pediatrician who understands working mothers. (Refer to the section on selecting a pediatrician before going on the initial interview.)

One last word of advice, make arrangements early with those who will be truly helpful to you when you first arrive home with the baby. Accept all help that is offered, and don't be afraid to delegate jobs to anyone who offers.

During your first days at home with your baby, don't get dressed! Lounging in a nice gown and robe will allow you to look nice, but you won't be tempted to venture out too soon. Enjoy your baby for a while before you start back into routines.

Be careful not to be the only one who attends to your baby's needs. Accept help from others, and allow your baby to feel comfortable with someone else. Allow your husband to begin his relationship with the baby. Like you, a dad has the right to learn, by trial and error, the things that work best for the baby.

During the latter part of your leave, double some of your recipes and freeze half of what is cooked so that those first few nights after work you can concentrate on the baby, not on meal preparation. Also, be sure you are staying in touch with your confidante at work. This will ease your transition back into the job.

Should you change your plans about returning to work, be sure that it is the best plan for your family, not because someone has made you feel guilty about working. You will have mixed feelings about returning to work, but only your and your partner can decide what is best . Start by asking yourself the following questions:

• How do you feel about sharing the care of your baby with a qualified caregiver?
• Do you really want to be an at-home mom?
• What does your intuition tell you is best for your baby?
• Can you survive on one income?
• Will you have enough insurance for the family on just your husband's benefits?

Before going back to work, the two of you should discuss how to divide household responsibilities. This would be a good time to list priorities. Include all of the activities that are necessary to make your lives run well. List such things as quality time with your child, housework, preparing meals, shopping, job performance, etc. Then adjust the list accordingly to emphasize the things that are important to both of you. Be flexible as you set up the housekeeping schedules; decide what has to be done, who is responsible for it, and when it will be completed, but know that changes may occur. Keep working with it until your family establishes a good routine.

Arrange to return to work on a Wednesday or Thursday, instead of a Monday; that way you will not have to confront the whole week immediately. Be careful not to show pictures of your baby all of the time; only show them if the person is genuinely interested. Never use your new motherhood role as an excuse for not completing an assignment, and never feel that you have to apologize for being a mother.

Breastfeeding Menu Plans

The following menu plans are designed to give your baby a healthy start, as well as give yourself a healthy recovery from pregnancy.

DAY 1

BREAKFAST	3/4 cup unsweetened cereal
	1 cup skim milk
	1 yellow peach
SNACK	1 1/2 cups low fat cottage cheese
	2 slices of pineapple
LUNCH	2 slices of whole wheat bread, not light variety
	3 slices turkey breast, fat free is okay
	1 slice Swiss or cheddar cheese, not American
	lettuce, tomato, mustard
	1 cup strawberries, fresh or frozen
SNACK	6 whole wheat crackers
DINNER	1 cup Chicken Stroganoff*
	1 cup wild rice
	1 1/2 cups steamed green beans
SNACK	1 1/2 cups low fat frozen yogurt

A mother is a mother still, The holiest thing alive.

– Coleridge

DAY 2

BREAKFAST
1 whole wheat English muffin with
  all fruit jam
1 cup skim milk or 1 cup low
  fat yogurt

SNACK
1 bran muffin, no butter
1 apple

LUNCH
Chef's salad:
  2 cups or more—lettuce, tomato,
    cucumber, carrots
  2 slices 98% fat free ham, chopped
  1 slice turkey, chopped
  2 slices Swiss or cheddar, chopped
3 Tablespoons low fat dressing*
6 whole wheat crackers

SNACK
  3 graham cracker squares
  1 cup skim milk

DINNER
  2 - 4 ounces Oranged Pork Fillets*
  1 baked sweet potato with
    imitation butter sprinkles
  1 cup cole slaw*
  1 roll

SNACK
  1 cup low fat frozen yogurt

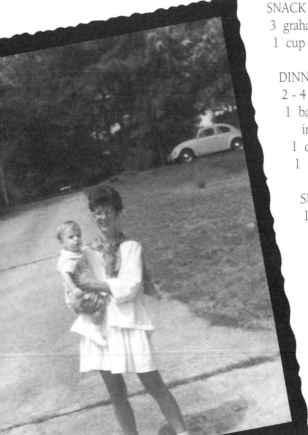

Day 3

BREAKFAST
: 3/4 cup unsweetened cereal
1 cup skim milk
1/2 cup strawberries

SNACK
: 1/2 English muffin topped with
2 Tablespoons pizza sauce
2 Tablespoons low fat, part skim mozzarella cheese

LUNCH
: 1 whole wheat pita
2 slices turkey
1 slice cheese
2 Tablespoons Cucumber Sauce*
1/2 cantaloupe

SNACK
: 1 1/2 cups low fat cottage cheese
2 slices pineapple

DINNER
: 1 cup spaghetti sauce with meat or vegetables
(rinse meat before adding to sauce)
1 cup pasta
1 tossed salad with low fat dressing*
1 roll

SNACK
: 1 cup low fat frozen yogurt

Day 4

BREAKFAST
: 1 whole wheat English muffin with all-fruit jam
1 cup skim milk

SNACK
: 1 banana

LUNCH
: 1 3/4 cup low fat cottage cheese
1/2 cantaloupe
1/2 strawberries
1 slice whole wheat bread
1 slice Swiss or cheddar melted on top

SNACK	3 graham cracker squares 1 cup skim milk

DINNER	2 Chicken Enchiladas* 1/2 cup Spanish rice* 1/2 cup fat-free refried beans

SNACK	1 cup low fat frozen yogurt

Day 5

BREAKFAST	3/4 cup unsweetened cereal 1 cup skim milk 1 peach

SNACK	3 graham cracker squares 1 cup calcium-added orange juice

LUNCH	2 slices whole wheat bread 3 slices turkey 1 slice Swiss or cheddar cheese lettuce, tomato, mustard 1 orange

SNACK	1 apple

DINNER	1 cup Chicken A La King* 1 cup pasta or rice 1 1/2 cups spinach salad with Honey Mustard dressing*

SNACK	1 cup low fat frozen yogurt

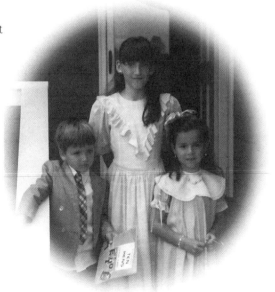

DAY 6

BREAKFAST	1 whole wheat English muffin with all-fruit spread 1 cup skim milk
SNACK	3 graham cracker squares 1 banana
LUNCH	1 foot-long French bread loaf, sliced in half, lengthwise; spread with: 1/4 cup pizza sauce per side 1/2 cup Mozzarella cheese any vegetable toppings you like
SNACK	1 peach
DINNER	1 6-ounce grilled steak, all visible fat removed before grilling 1 Twice Baked Potato* 1 1/2 cup Marinated Broccoli Salad*
SNACK	1 cup low fat frozen yogurt

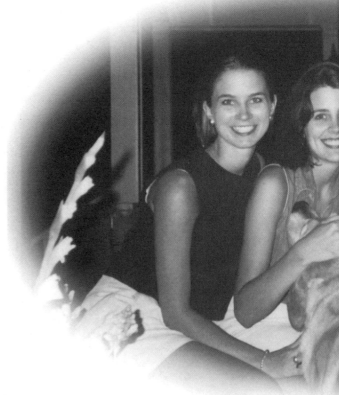

Day 7

BREAKFAST	3/4 cup unsweetened cereal 1 cup skim milk 1 peach
SNACK	1 banana
LUNCH	Chef's Salad (same as Day 2) 6 whole wheat crackers
SNACK	3 graham cracker squares 1 apple
DINNER	Low Country Boil* : 1 cup shrimp, 1 piece of sausage, 1 corn, 2 potatoes 1 cup spinach salad with Honey Mustard dressing*
SNACK	1 cup low fat frozen yogurt

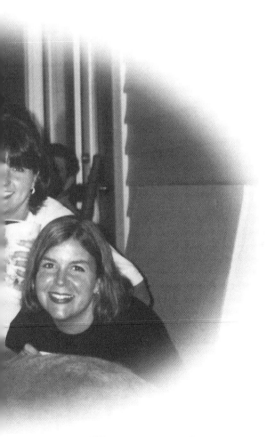

Each friend represents a world in us, a world possibly not born until they arrive, and it is only by this meeting that a new world is born.

– Anais Nin

Parenting

Parenting is difficult. The rewards seem high on good days, and hard to find on bad days. As you are in the trenches of everyday parenting, remind yourself that you are doing your best. Any decision you have made previously was what you deemed to be best at that time. Since you cannot change the past, look ahead to the future.

Remember that children learn best by example, so model appropriate behavior. Know that each child is truly different. You must spend time with each one before you truly appreciate their differences, and be able to adjust individual discipline accordingly. A parent who administers discipline with love and acceptance will have a secure child. Encourage creativity and optimism.

During the first year of your child's life, use a basic infant care and development book. Spend time getting to know your child. Once you have gotten to know your child's personality and your style of parenting, choose one or more of the following books to keep on hand for guidance.

It is more blessed to give than to receive.

– Acts 20:35

American Academy of Pediatrics. *Caring For Your Baby And Young Child,* and *Caring For Your School-Age Child.* Bantam Books, 1995.

Brazelton, T. Berry. *Touchpoints.* Addison-Wesley, 1992.

DeFrancis, Beth. *The Parents Resource Almanac.* Bob Adams, Inc., 1994.

Eisenberg, Arlene; Murkoff, Heidi; and Hathaway, Sandee. *What To Expect When You're Expecting; What To Expect The First Year;* and *What To Expect The Toddler Years.* Workman Publishing, 1994.

Favaro, Peter. *Smart Parenting.* Nightingale-Conant Corporation, 1994.

Gootman, Marilyn. *The Loving Parents Guide To Discipline.* Berkley Books, 1995.

Koch, JoAnne and Freeman, Linda. *Good Parents For Hard Times.* Simon & Schuster, 1992.

Smalley, Gary and Trent, John. *The Blessing.* Pocket Books, 1986.

Spock, Benjamin. *Dr. Spock's Baby and Child Care, 6th edition.* Penguin Books, 1992.

White, Burton. *The New First Three Years Of Life,* and *Raising A Happy, Unspoiled Child.*

Woititz, Janet. *Healthy Parenting.* Simon & Schuster, 1992.

Zigler, Zig. *Raising Positive Kids In A Negative World.* Simon & Schuster, 1995.

STRIVING FOR EQUAL PARENTING

Although dads today pitch in more, do they really pull their fair share in parenting? If you ask most moms, the answer is "No!" Although most dads do spend more time with their children, most of that time is spent doing things that are fun. When it comes down to the actual "parenting," the weight falls on the mother's shoulders. Jobs like menu planning, grocery shopping, scheduling doctor's appointments, buying school clothes, planning birthday parties, signing up for extra activities (dance lessons, Little League, Scouts, etc.), pick up/ drop off for extra activities, being a room mother or Scout leader, helping with homework, picking up prescriptions, giving out medication, breaking up sibling fights, nurturing, and more, all are a part of being a mom.

Many husbands today do take a bigger share of traditionally "mom" jobs. In order to encourage your husband to participate more in parenting, begin using these suggestions early in your child's life.

Allow your husband to learn through trial and error what really helps when calming your baby. If you give him the time and space to figure out his own techniques, the more confidence he will have, and the more he'll do.

When you ask your husband to help out with a job, be precise about the help you need.

Once the job is completed, don't criticize his effort. The less monitoring and criticism your husband receives for his effort with parenting and housework, the more likely he is to continue his efforts.

Make a short list of the jobs for him to do that will help you. Once you've given him the list, be patient, and expect him to comply.

If you are expecting your first child, you may not realize how important it will be to your family to have equal parenting. By truly sharing the responsibilities, your life will run more smoothly.

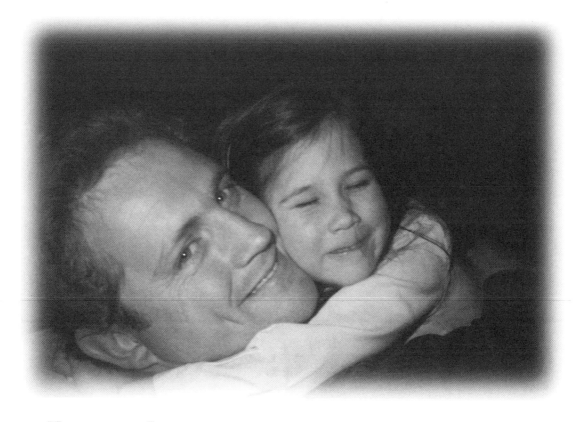

Love and Care For Your Premature Infant

A premature baby is born before the 36th week of pregnancy. In most cases, the cause of pre-term labor is unknown. Due to advanced medical knowledge and technique, however, a preemie born today has a much better chance of survival.

As the parent of a pre-term infant, you should be aware of the following:

Your baby may be skinny (because there is not much fat under the skin); have reddish or translucent skin with visible arteries and veins; may have lanugo (a fine layer of body hair); and may not be physically developed.

Your baby will begin to look more like a full-term infant as he begins to reach the original due date (the 40-week mark).

You should talk to, touch, and hold your baby as soon as possible. This will comfort both of you.

Try to breastfeed if at all possible. By nature your milk is formulated to meet your infant's needs and breastfeeding will make a beneficial difference in your baby's progress.

Become part of the "team" in the special care nursery. Ask questions and let the nurses know that you want to be part of team that cares for your newborn.

If you go home before your baby does, spend as much time as possible each day with your baby in the special care nursery. Do allow yourself some rest time so that you will be ready for the homecoming. Bring in family pictures and soft stuffed toys to decorate your baby's area. Most special care nurseries will have your baby's name on her bed, make sure her name is used often.

You will need an infant car seat for baby's ride home. Make sure it meets safety standards and will accommodate your baby's smaller size. Devices to secure your baby's head in the seat are available at most baby accessories stores. Be sure there is nothing between the back of the baby's head and neck and the car seat.

Bouncy seats and swings may be harmful to baby's delicate respiratory system; check with your pediatrician before purchasing either piece of equipment.

Your baby will probably feed frequently, since he can only take in small amounts of milk at a time. Be patient and allow yourself to really enjoy each feeding as a bonding time. You may also need to keep your house a little warmer.

As you begin to track your baby's development, remember to use the corrected age (his original due date) and know that all children develop at their own rate.

Caring For Your
Special Needs Child

As parents, we should all try to do everything we can for each child. This becomes more prevalent when you have a special needs child. You will be expected to make many different decisions concerning your child's care and well being. When faced with major decisions with regard to your child, contemplate the following.

• You must always follow your intuition as to what is best for your child. You must trust that each decision was the best choice at the time it was made.

• Approach every part of your child's life with the hopes of achieving what is best for your child.

• Be an advocate for your child.

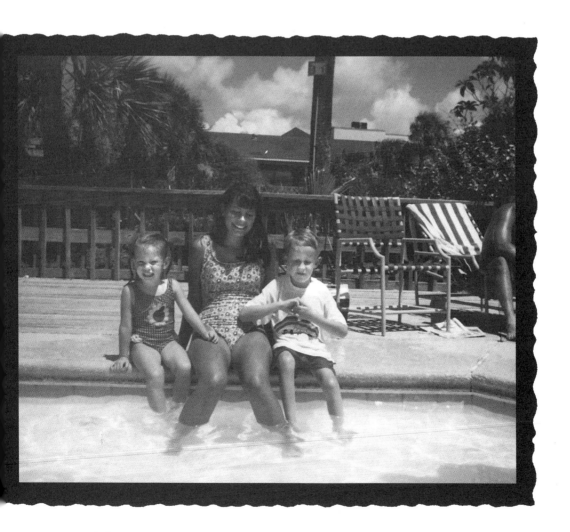

Listen to advice and
accept instruction, that
you may gain wisdom for
the future.

– Proverbs 19:20

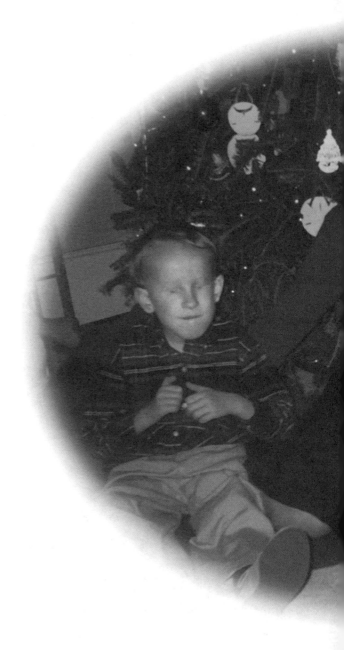

• Seek support. Contact agencies or groups through your pediatrician or local
health department. Try to network with other parents who have children with
similar needs.
• Do all that you can, but remember, you are only one person. You are not
super mom.
• You must not neglect your other children's needs or your own.

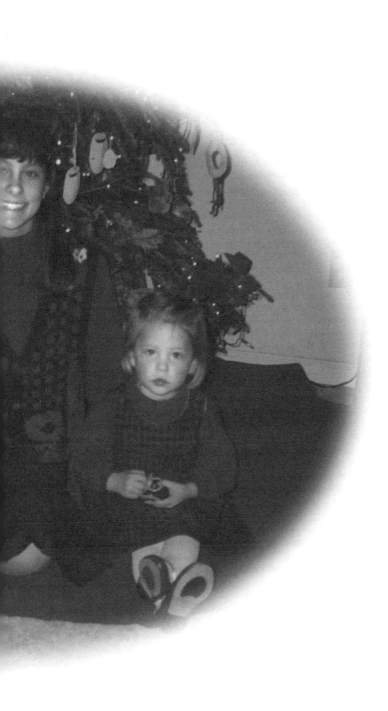

SUGGESTED READINGS:

Albrecht, Donna. *Raising A Child Who Has A Physical Disability.* John Wiley & Sons, Inc., 1995.

Batshaw, Mark. *Your Child Has A Disability.* Little, Brown, & Company, 1991.

Rosner, Jerome. *Helping Children Overcome Learning Difficulties.* Walker & Company, 1993.

Touray, Sandy and Wilson-Portuondo, Maria. *Helping Your Special Needs Child.* Prima Publishing, 1995.

Can You Really Spoil Your Newborn?

Some of the old wives' tales we have been told for generations include: "If you pick up your baby every time she cries, you will spoil her" or "That baby has already learned to manipulate you." Both statements are false.

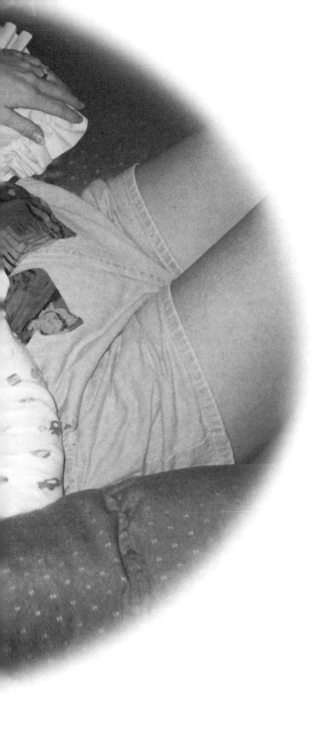

F
rom small
beginnings come
great things.

– Proverb

A newborn only cries when she needs something: a diaper change, a feeding, or to be held. By quickly responding to your baby when she cries, you let her know that someone will react to her needs, thus encouraging a more secure baby. As far as manipulation, a newborn cannot maneuver you to do anything.

As a mother, you should hold, rock, talk to, sing to, and read to your baby often. These actions will produce a more secure infant, who will thus be ready to tackle the next stage of development.

Multiple Births

You don't know whether to laugh or cry: you have just found out that you are expecting more than one baby. Due to advanced medical treatments for infertility, multiple births are on the rise. (Traditionally, about two in every one hundred births will be a multiple birth.)

You may feel disappointed and/or scared; you are not alone. This is very alarming news for many families. The key to getting through this pregnancy, the impending birth, as well as the first year of parenting multiples, will be the preparations made.

During the pregnancy, discomforts will be even more intense. Keep an ongoing list of discomfort symptoms and questions that you can ask your physician during your frequent visits. Plan on more prenatal visits with a multiple pregnancy, and heed all of your physician's recommendations. Some questions to address early in the pregnancy include:

How can I best meet my increased nutritional demands?

When should I stop working?

What additional testing will I need?

How many additional ultrasounds are necessary?

Do you have any former patients who have delivered multiples whom I could contact for support, as well as advice?

You may be confined to bed during the last stages of your pregnancy. Begin to make preparations early on so that your family can survive without your income. If you already have one or more children, arrange for help with their care, and keep them abreast of what is occurring during different stages of the pregnancy. Children usually react better if they have some idea about what to expect.

As you begin to prepare for two or more infants in your home, you will need to double up on some equipment. For example, you will need two car seats, two beds, two high chairs, and double the number of diapers. Prior to arriving home with the babies, divide household responsibilities with your spouse, and know that you will only be able to do what is necessary. Purchase paper plates, and have the numbers of some of your favorite restaurant delivery services handy.

When you first arrive home, keep good records. In a notebook, list who was fed when and how much, bath schedules, medications, etc. At first, this will be the only way to keep up with the daily details. If one baby is up at night, wake the other... then maybe you can sleep when they are sleeping.

Spend time during daily routines to get to know both babies. Even though they are twins, or more, each is also an individual. Appreciate the differences, and encourage the closeness that multiples usually share. Remember, the first few months are the roughest, but you will learn to cope.

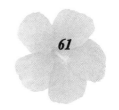

SUGGESTED READINGS:

Friedrich, Elizabeth and Rowland, Cherry. *Parents Guide To Raising Twins*. St. Martins Press, 1983.

Noble, Elizabeth. *Having Twins*. Houghton-Mifflin Company, 1991.

Norothy, Pamela Patrick. *Joy Of Twins*. Crown Trade Paperbacks, 1993.

Finding Good Child Care

One of the most critical decisions you will make is who will care for your child when you return to work. This decision will no only affect your transition back to work, but it will also have an impact on your child's quality of life.

Begin early in your quest for quality child care. If this is your first baby, begin your search during pregnancy. Allow yourself ample time to find the center or home-care situation that will best meet your family's needs. Many people spend less time selecting a child care center than they do choosing a new car. Don't just pick a number a number out of the Yellow Pages, use the following information to your advantage.

The following guidelines will assist you in your search for quality care, as well as present sample questions to ask, and a checklist to take with you on your visits. *A preferred center or home-care situation will offer:*

- a stable staff;
- small groups of children;
- proper attention according to the child's developmental stage;
- developmentally appropriate activities;
- encouragement of parental involvement.

Once you have found centers/homes that meet the foregoing criteria, proceed to the next set of guidelines.

- Visit at least two or more centers/homes.
- Take somebody with you, preferably your spouse. Two reactions are better than one.
- Consider your first impression to be valuable. If it just doesn't feel right when you first arrive, follow your instincts.
- Allow plenty of time for the visit.
- Be wary of a center that does not allow drop-in visits by parents. A center may may mention a specific time when you can observe the children engaged in activities.
- Meet with the center's director and the caregiver for your baby.
- Have a list of questions ready to ask the person who will be caring for your child.
- Spend at least one hour observing the area where your child will be placed.
- Ask for references, or the phone numbers of some of the parents who have children currently in the program.

Make a list of what is most important to you regarding your child's care. The following examples show the difference between what is developmentally appropriate for an infant as well as a preschooler:

INFANT

1. Baby is talked to during feeding and diapering.
2. Baby is responded to quickly.
3. Baby is appropriately stimulated.
4. Baby is not left in one place all day, such as his/her bed.

PRESCHOOLER

1. Creativity is valued by the caregiver.
2. Child is given the opportunity to choose from suitable options.
3. Child has meaningful play experiences.
4. The classroom has flexibility so that questions are answered, and the children help define the direction.

These next questions may help you select the right place for your child:

How do you handle a baby who cries persistently?

Can my child bring her favorite stuffed toy from home?

What would a typical day be like for my child?

How can I be involved as a parent?

What could a baby/child do that would really make you angry? How would you handle that situation? (Look for age-appropriate answers to this question. For example, I would be wary of a toddler's caregiver who gets angry at toileting accidents, but I would feel more confident with one who said that she will not tolerate a child hurting another child, so she provides a "break from the group" for the child who has lost his self-control.)

What is your background with children?

How long have you been an employee/caregiver? (Look for a center with a low turnover rate; your child needs stability.)

CHILD CARE CHECKLIST

Yes	No	
		Center or home visited:
		Smoke-free environment
		Floors are clean/carpeted
		At least one adult is always present
		Electrical outlets are covered
		Toys are in good condition
		Toys are age appropriate
		Safe outdoor area
		Floor space not overcrowded
		Low adult/child ratio

NO PHYSICAL PUNISHMENT

Yes	No	
		Caregiver has sincere loving attitude toward children
		Children seem happy and content
		Secure evacuation plan
		Well-planned program with flexibility to allow for inquisitive children

INFANT NEEDS:

Yes	No	
		Crib for each baby
		Babies are not simply lying unresponsively in cribs
		Babies are talked to during feeding and diapering
		Babies seem stimulated
		Soft rattles, blocks, and balls
		Enough crawling space
		Mobiles and pictures for the babies' visual stimulation

GUIDELINES FOR SELECTING A NANNY OR IN-HOME SITTER

- Don't ignore your first impression.
- Allow plenty of time for the interview.
- Have a list of questions ready to ask.
- Check all references, even if the agency states that they have already checked them.
- Take someone with you on the interview.

(Once again, two reactions are better than one.)

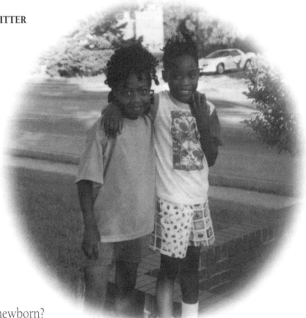

SAMPLE QUESTIONS

1. Why are you seeking an infant-care position?
2. What makes you suited for this type of work?
3. What type of training do you have?
4. For how long (or how limited) of a time would you be willing to work?
5. Tell me about your expertise in taking care of a newborn?
6. Do you have other responsibilities or any problems that could interfere with your work?
7. Where you have worked up until now?
8. May I talk with someone there?
9. How long were you there and why did you leave?
10. How would you handle a baby who cries persistently?

11. Do you think that a baby can be spoiled by picking her up every time she cries?

12. Have you had a physical examination, including a tuberculosis test, in the last six months?

QUESTIONS TO ASK THE AGENCY

1. How and where do you recruit your applicants?

2. How do you screen your applicants?

3. What will you do if the placement isn't satisfactory?

4. What are your fees? Do you charge an upfront fee? Is this refundable?

5. Can you give me the names and phone numbers of families in my area who have used your agency?

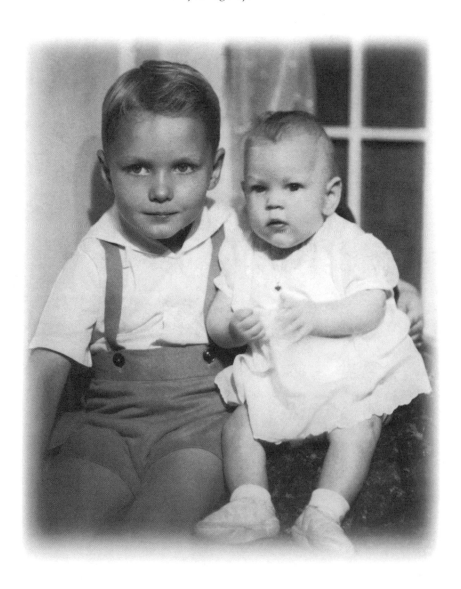

Selecting Your Baby's Pediatrician

Another responsibility best met during your pregnancy is the selection of a pediatrician. Most pediatricians now request, some even require, an interview prior to the delivery of your baby. If you do not choose a pediatrician before the delivery, you may be assigned one at the hospital. If you do not prefer the doctor you are assigned, it may be difficult to find a new one. When selecting a pediatrician, consider the following:

What are the doctor's credentials? Look for AAP (American Association of Pediatrics) and ABFP (American Board of Family Practitioners).

With what hospital is the doctor affiliated?

Where is the office located?

What are the office hours?

How are emergencies handled?

How are financial matters handled?

It is imperative that you establish a good relationship with your child's pediatrician. This will make a difference on how your child views doctors for a lifetime. *When you first visit the office, look for the following:*

- Is the waiting area relaxing, and are toys/books provided for the children?
- What is the average waiting time?
- Does the doctor's personality mesh with yours and your baby's?
- Does the doctor have similar views on child development?

On the initial interview, find out the pediatrician's position on the following:

- What are his/her views on working mothers?
- Does the doctor believe in preventative medicine?
- What is the office policy on returning phone calls?
- What is his/her views on infant and childhood nutrition?
- How often should you feed the baby?
- When should you add solids and how do you handle a picky toddler?
- When does the pediatrician feel the need to use antibiotics?

As with any of the service individuals your child will need to come in contact with during her lifetime, your approach will make a huge impact. It is essential that you assist your child in building quality relationships with her health care providers; this will encourage her to be an active participant in her health care as she matures.

If I have to, I can do anything.

– Helen Reddy

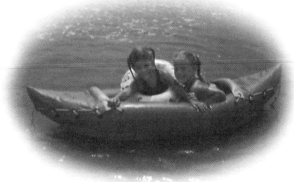

Preparing Your Child For A Sibling

When you brought your first child home from the hospital, you and your husband had to prepare yourselves for this new family member. You both had much to learn about baby care, parenting, and adjusting your lives to incorporate the baby.

Though you and your husband may feel very happy about the arrival of the new baby, your firstborn may have different feelings: anger, jealousy, or the fear of being replaced. These feelings may worsen when the new baby actually comes home to stay.

When you bring home your second child, you and your husband will be better prepared for this homecoming, but your firstborn child will need help making adjustments.

The best thing you can do is to relax. Children take their cues from what is going on around them, so if you are overly anxious, your child will be too. Here are some suggestions to help ease the transition.

Tell the child about the new baby early in the pregnancy, otherwise, he may sense that something is going on and being kept from him. (If you have a history of miscarriage, wait until the first twelve weeks have passed.)

Make any planned major changes early in the pregnancy. For example: toilet training, moving to a new home, new child care arrangements, or making the move from a crib to a bed. If the changes cannot be made at least one month before the new baby arrives, wait until the baby has been home for a couple of months before making the major change.

Find a book at the library or bookstore that shows the month-by-month development of the fetus. Age-appropriate books, which provide information on your child's level of understanding, are available.

Introduce your child to the new baby early with ultrasound pictures and/or videos. As soon as possible, begin calling the baby by name so that the older child realizes that this is who you are talking about. If you are going to keep the baby's sex a surprise, always refer to the baby as yours and ours, never just as my baby.

Try out names you've selected and let your older child help decide on the name for the baby.

Familiarize your child with babies in general. Look at pictures of her as a baby. Visit the hospital nursery if possible to see what a newborn looks like. If a friend has a baby, schedule a short visit. Point out any other babies you see during the day. Explain to your child that the baby will mostly sleep, eat, and cry in the beginning.

If your child is interested, involve him in some of the preparations. Decorating the nursery, going through his old baby items to decide what can be

Our happiness in this world depends on the affections we are enabled to inspire.

– Duchesse de Praslin

used by the new baby, allowing him to pick out a couple of inexpensive items for the baby's room, are all good ideas.

Help the child become accustomed to spending less time alone with you. Incorporate some firstborn/father special times, maybe a special breakfast out once a week, an afternoon at the park, or another planned weekly activity just for the two of them.

As the due date approaches, prepare your child for your hospital stay. Let her help you pack—ask for something to take along that belongs to her (to keep you company). A picture of her, a teddy bear, or some of her artwork, will help you both to feel connected.

Help your older child get used to riding in the back seat in the car. If you have dual air bags, both children will ride in the back; if not, the baby will be safer in the front with you, in a rear-facing infant seat.

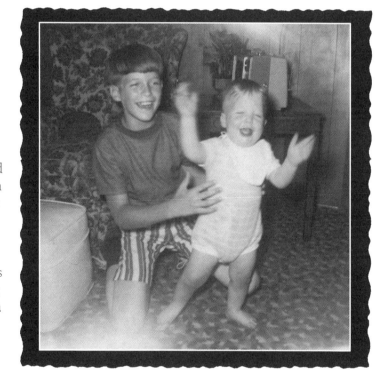

Buy several small surprises for younger children. Wrap them individually, and put them away. Each time someone comes to visit with a gift for the new baby, bring out one of these gifts for your toddler.

Before the delivery, take your child to pick out a "gift" for the baby. He can bring this to the hospital for their first meeting.

Select and wrap a small gift for your older child and take it to the hospital. When the older sibling comes to visit, give her the gift from the baby, which will help to start things out on a positive note.

When the child comes to visit in the hospital, do not have the baby in the room when the older child arrives.

Allow your child to greet you privately, then introduce the newborn. (This way the older child is not threatened that his place with you is being challenged.) Give your firstborn some jobs that only a big brother or big sister could do: getting diapers, pulling out the individual wipes, or picking out an outfit.

With close supervision, allow your firstborn to touch and maybe even hold the baby. Depending on the age and maturity of your firstborn, she may be able to help with feedings, burping the baby, or bath time. (Never leave a child under the age of 12 with full responsibility for the baby.)

Don't overdo the preparation. Remember, your older child still has other interests in his life, and that the adjustment will take time.

Separation From Mother

During your child's early years, an occasion may arise when you will have to be separated from your child. This will most likely occur when you are in the hospital having the second child, but whatever the reason, the following tips may help your youngster through the separation.

Allow the child to sleep with something that belongs to you. Usually a nylon gown is a favorite. For toddlers, this same item may be carried around during the day for security.

Try to keep your child's routine as close to normal as possible. Young children are creatures of habit, and a routine will offer needed security during this separation.

When you do have the opportunity to talk to your child, make sure that she knows you are listening. Try repeating the last sentence, or word if this is a very young child; this will reassure your child that what she has to say is important, and that you are listening to her. Encourage the caregiver and your spouse to do the same thing.

Use some of your child's artwork to decorate your room. This will help both of you to feel connected.

The child should be given continuous reassurance that you will be coming back; he can never hear that too much!

Single Parenting

Most of us would agree that the best environment in which to raise a child is in a household of two loving, involved parents. The reality is that many households are run by a committed single parent, determined to offer the best for her child. Because the stress of parenthood is certain to be magnified when facing it by yourself, these next suggestions may be useful.

Encourage your child to have an endearing relationship with a male whom 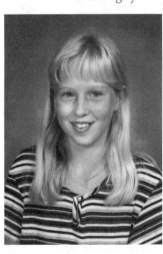 you trust and respect. This may be your father, a close friend, your minister, or your brother. Children need good relationships with adults of both sexes.

Get together with another single mom and trade off babysitting: once a month, one keeps the children, while the other gets a night off. You can also go on outings together, have some meals together, and support each other. In turn, this will give your child a playmate and friend.

Plan some holiday get-togethers with other families. This will help your child to understand the importance of close relationships.

Remind yourself that you are doing your best. Seek people who are supportive, and associate with them.

Get involved in family-oriented organizations, such as churches and Scouts.
Make special time for your child.

Be optimistic. Keep the past in the past, and look forward to the future.

SUGGESTED READINGS:

Boyd, Julia; Hogan, Linda; Kingsolver, Barbara; Lamott,Anne; and Moseley-Brown, Carol. *The Single Mother's Companion*. Seal Press, 1994.

Engber, Andrea and Klunghess, Leah. *The Complete Single Mother*. Adams Publishing, 1995.

StepParenting

One of the many types of families in our current society is the blended family, which combines different families through a marriage, with one or both parents becoming a stepparent. The responsibility of being a stepparent brings with it many transitions as well as obstacles to face.

The stepparent who is married to the custodial parent faces many challenges. The couple, the children, and the relationship between parent and child will change. The way the adults involved handle these demands will affect the entire family. Here are some suggestions if you are the stepparent in the household.

Discuss the rules, the discipline style, the routine, and any other aspect of day-to-day life with your partner. It is imperative to discuss with your spouse beforehand any form of discipline you may eventually administer.

In the beginning, and until sound relationships have been formed, it is important that you support the custodial parent. Any disagreements with the way a situation is being handled should be discussed privately.

Take the opportunity to build trust in a timeframe that is mapped out by the child and the custodial parent. This is not the time for you to recommend your "better way" of doing things.

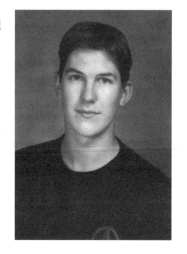

Allow time to get to know the child and for the child to get to know you. Take time to listen to the child, and plan simple activities that you both will enjoy.

There are also relationship adjustments that will occur if you are married to a non-custodial parent with visitation privileges. The following preparations have helped me during my ongoing education in how to be an effective stepparent:

Encourage the father to be a parent to the child, not just a buddy. It is easy for a non-custodial father to feel pressure to be a "good time" dad, out of guilt. Although this may seem to be what the children want, children feel more secure when they live with limits. This facilitates a stable environment in which he is allowed to be the type of parent he should.

Make plans together for the visit. Where will you go, when and what you will eat, who will be responsible for what, when is bedtime, etc. Preparation and information help to provide that needed security, and as a couple you will be equipped to relax and enjoy the children.

Children deserve unconditional love, and this is what you must offer. No matter what, they must know that they are loved and accepted by the non-custodial parent, and as the stepparent, this will be rewarding to your life also.

Unconditional love may best be obtained by learning to "let go." One weekend a month, every six months, or even less, is not the time to push what you deem as a better lifestyle on his children. The time will be better spent getting to know each other, having fun together, and making wonderful memories. Before making an issue out of anything, ask yourself, "Will this even be remembered in five days, five weeks, or five years from now?" Is it worth putting a strain on your relationship? The answer probably will be no.

SUGGESTED READINGS:

Berman, Claire. *Making It As A Step Parent.* Harper & Row, 1986.
Kaufman, Taube. *The Combined Family.* Pelnum Press, 1993.
Lofas, Jeannette with Sova, Dawn. *Step Parenting: Everything You Need To Know To Make It Work.* Kensington Books, 1995.
Prilik, Pearl Ketover. *The Art Of Step-Mothering.* WRS Publishing, 1994.

Staying Sane While You Stay At Home

The decision to stay home with your baby is one of the most important choices you will ever make. The love and attention your baby will receive from you is the best gift you can give your child. Although children who are in a quality child care situation will also thrive and grow up to be happy, well-adjusted adults, no one will attend to your child in the same way that you will. Even though you know that this is for the best, there are times when you may question your decision, and your self-esteem may ebb.

Many people in our society will question why a smart woman would want to stay home. You may feel isolated, unappreciated, and depressed.

When you are at home, you don't receive a paycheck, you don't have other adults to converse with daily, and you are not praised by a superior or co-worker for the good job you are doing. You may question your parenting skills, and wonder if staying home is the best decision.

To make the most of your decision to stay at home, try some of these suggestions.

• Get out of the house with your child daily. Take your stroller downtown or to the mall and walk around. You and your baby will enjoy seeing other people and sights, plus hearing new sounds. This will give you the opportunity to get out of the house and get some needed fresh air.

• Seek out other stay-at-home moms and get together. This will provide you with adult interaction, support from others who have made the same decision you have, and playmates for your child.

• Consider doing some type of volunteer work one afternoon a week.

• You do not have to spend every minute with your baby; a mother with a healthy self-esteem will be a better mother, so take some time for yourself.

• Consider hiring a teenager occasionally for a couple of hours to give yourself a break.

• Start a baby-sitting co-op. Each member begins with the same number of "bills," each worth 30 minutes of sitting time. This a good way to insure that everyone gets a fair share of sitting time and time out.

• Don't be a SUPER MOM. Ask for help and seek support.

• Encourage your husband to have special times with your child; this will help to build their relationship, and provide you with a needed break.

Take advantage of local resources:

• Go to the library once a week. Involve your child in story hours, puppet shows, and the selection of books, and take the time to find some interesting books for yourself.

• Get to know your local parks, museums, or other points of interest.

• Check to see if there is a local mother's center or at-home mother's support group; if not, start one!

• For those on a budget, seek out local consignment shops for quality pre-owned clothes, toys, books, and equipment at very reasonable prices.

• Check with some of your local churches to see which "Mother's Morning Out" program is best for you. Certain day care centers offer part-time drop-offs with prior notification.

Another valuable resource is *Welcome Home*, a magazine written by at-home moms, for at-home moms. It is published by Mothers At Home, 8310A Old Courthouse Road, Vienna, VA 22182.

Handling Working Mom Guilt

There are many reasons that women work today. The majority of moms that I know either work because their family needs the income for survival, or the insurance package to help provide for their family's health care. Whatever the motivation is for your decision to work, you inevitably will experience times of the dreaded "mommy guilt." One way to help combat these feelings is to make a list of the advantages to being a working mother.

You are lucky to have a job that enables you to provide for your child.

Receiving a paycheck, a raise, or a compliment from a superior, helps to increase your self- esteem. A woman with high self-esteem is a better mother.

Working mothers provide daughters with wonderful role models.

Dividing the household responsibilities will help your children learn that it takes the whole family's participation to make the home run smoothly. This is especially beneficial for sons, since they probably will be part of a dual-career family when they marry.

In a quality child-care situation, your child is gaining valuable skills, such as the ability to get along with peers and take direction from another adult.

There always will be the debate about whether it is better for you to stay home with your children or to work outside of the home. Because there are benefits to both sides, what is important is that you do all you can to be happy in your situation. The following suggestions have been helpful in my quest to balance all of my roles.

Get up thirty minutes earlier each morning during the work week. Get yourself ready first, then take fifteen minutes to snuggle with your child. (We like to sit in the recliner and watch cartoons.) This special time together seems to set the tone for the day. The other fifteen minutes is so that you don't have to rush around to leave on time; this will also help to start the day off right. If you have more than one child, divide your week to accommodate each child; then spend ten minutes each evening reconnecting with each of them.

At least once a week I go to a social lunch with a friend or co-workers. I consider this to be a wise use of my time, since I benefit from time well spent with a friend, and I am not taking additional time away from my family.

Evaluate your priorities and then relax your standards where applicable. For example, I value quality time with my child more than an immaculate home; therefore, I have relaxed my standards regarding housework, thus affording me extra time with my family.

Take care of yourself. If you are worn out, stressed out , or overwhelmed, you will not be as effective as a parent. You must take care of yourself physically and emotionally.

Strive to enjoy a well-balanced diet, and be sure to exercise daily. I often incorporate time with my child with my exercise time. I may pull him in his wagon as I go for a walk, or we may run up the big hill at the park, then slide down in a box over the pinestraw. As a working mom, it is emotionally healing to preserve at least one hour a week just for yourself. This time may be spent in an exercise class, painting class, cooking class, reading at the library, or any other activity you enjoy. Taking this time for yourself will help to rejuvenate you for the demanding role of being a working mom.

Seek support from those who are truly understanding. Try some of the other mothers with whom you work, or if your mother worked outside of the home, she may have some good advice.

SUGGESTED READINGS:

Lague, Louise. *The Working Mom's Book Of Hints, Tips, And Everyday Wisdom.* Peterson's, 1995.

Norris, Gloria and Miller, Jo Ann. *The Working Mother's Complete Handbook.* Plume Books, 1984.

It is necessary to try to surpass one's self always; this occupation ought to last as long as life.

– Queen Christina of Sweden

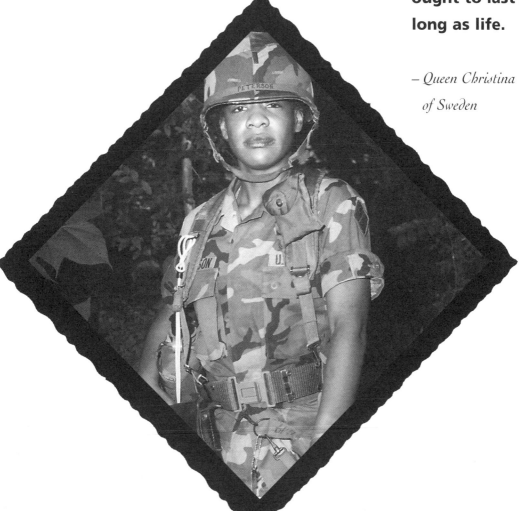

Leaving The House On Time

Leave a basket by the back door to fill with things that you need to take with you in the mornings: your child's diaper bag or book bag, special signed forms for school, your calendar/date book, or anything else you must have. Keep your keys in the same place (a hook, for instance) to eliminate the hassle of having to search for them.

Get out everyone's clothes the night before, and make sure any last-minute ironing is already done. Make sure that lunches are prepared or lunch money is out and ready to go. Plan lunches that can be made the night before, and still be palatable the next day. As your children get older, ask them what kinds of things they enjoy most for lunch. Have some of their favorites available, then let each child be responsible for his/her own lunch. (You will find that lunches are more likely to be eaten if the child fixes his/her own.) Pack the diaper bag the night before, and make sure all extras are included.

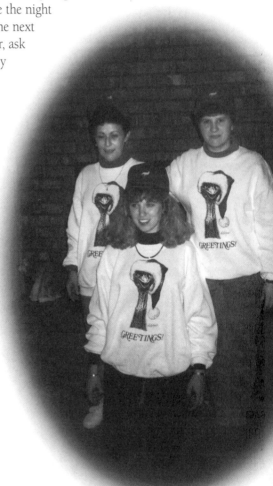

Set up an emergency changing station for that last-minute accident that always happens just as you are leaving the house.

Have breakfast items ready: cereal with milk, a banana, whole wheat toast or a bagel, and fruit juice will help to make a good start for the day.

To be social is to be forgiving.

– Robert Frost

Transforming Car Time Into Quality Time

As a busy mom, it becomes necessary to reconstruct some of the everyday routine into quality time with your family. The time spent traveling to and from work/ school/ child care is a prime example of such a time. One of my mom's best argument-enders was to prevent anyone from saying another word until you pointed out at least five good things you saw on the drive. This little trick worked wonders.

Use the time to really connect with your child. On the way to school/child care/work, discuss the day's plans—who will pick up your child, any events occurring after work, what activity they are looking forward to at school, what's for lunch—any of the little things that will complete the day. On the way home, ask lead-in questions such as, "Who did you play with today?" or "What did you do today?"

Invent silly games. One of our favorites is the Sound Effect Game. We take turns asking each other to make distinct sounds: wind whistling through the trees, baby birds crying for dinner, a fire engine racing to a fire, a baseball bat hitting the ball. Your child/children will love being creative.

Sing silly songs. These may include songs you know, or ones that you invent.

Play the rhyming game. One person says a word, then the other has to say a rhyming word.

The old standards like I Spy take on a new meaning when you first teach them to your children.

Menu Planning For Busy Families

As parents of young children, parts of our lives are very hectic. But one section that can be simplified is meal time, which should be one of the most enjoyable parts of the day. Some of the best memories made occur during the family's dinner time. The opportunity for children to test new ideas, for parents to help socialize the family, and the chance just to be together, are all important aspects of meal time.

As a working mother, I know how chaotic a family's schedule can be. Trying to coordinate everyone's agenda so that you can all be together at dinner may be next to impossible. Instead, set your dinner time, and then don't schedule anything that will conflict with it. Your children need the stability of a set family meal time, and the positive impact it will have on their social and emotional development is priceless. If it is impossible to plan a family dinner time for every night of the week, make sure that you set aside several nights of the week. This extra effort will be worth it to your family.

One of the culprits that can hinder an enjoyable meal together is the power struggle between parent and child over eating a balanced meal. As parents, it is imperative that we offer healthy choices to our children, and to children it is essential that the food taste good. To satisfy both parties, plan menus that are nutritious and delicious.

Another barrier to an enjoyable meal with the family is having the time to shop for and prepare it. This becomes increasingly demanding when squeezed into a busy lifestyle. By designing menus that are easy to buy for, as well as simple to make, offering wholesome meals becomes less complicated. Another plus to designing simple meals is the opportunity for your children to help with preparation. This is a great time management technique, since you combine quality time with your children, the option of teaching food preparation techniques, and you get the meal made!

The way food is served can be just as important as what is served when young children are involved. Offering foods that are easy for little hands to manage will be a plus. Make sure that foods are small enough to prevent choking hazards; all round foods should be halved. Serve appropriate portions to your little ones by following these guidelines: serve toddlers and preschoolers about one tablespoon of food for each year of age; include two to three servings of meat/protein, four servings from the dairy group, three vegetables, and three fruits, and at least six servings of grains/breads each day. Sample servings include: 1/2 piece of fruit, 1/2 slice of bread, 1/2 cup yogurt, or 1/2 of a 3-ounce burger. Offering a good variety will be the key, but remember, a child may need to be presented with a certain food numerous times before she will even try it.

These menus were designed to be family friendly and the recipes are simple. This will also help in promoting meal preparation tasks that children can do.

MENUS

Baked Georgia Chicken*	Shake 'em Up Pork Chops*
Cheesy Potatoes*	Macaroni and Cheese*
Green Beans	Snow Peas with Mushrooms
Biscuits	Italian Bread Slices

Bar-B-Que Chicken (baked or grilled)	
Slim and Thin Fries*	Vegetarian Chili*
Lemon Broccoli*	Fresh Fruit with Yogurt Topping
60 Minute Rolls*	Corn Muffins*

It is better to decide between our enemies than our friends; for one of our friends will most likely become our enemy; but on the other hand, one of your enemies will probably become your friend.

– Bias

Crunchy Herb Fish* Chicken Pot Pie*
Sautéed Summer Squash Sweet & Sour Broccoli Salad*
Honey Baby Carrots* Hot Spiced Peaches*
Wheat Rolls Mini French Bread Loaves
Quick and Easy Low Country Boil* Garden Salad

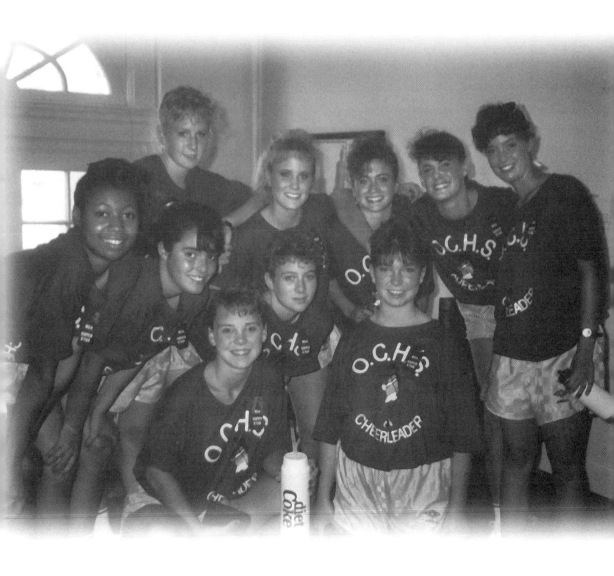

Adolescent Menu Plans

Day 1

BREAKFAST	1 bagel
	all-fruit jam
	1 cup skim milk
	1 banana
SNACK	6 graham cracker squares
	1 apple
LUNCH	Chef's salad:
	lettuce, tomato, cucumber, carrots
	1/2 cup sharp cheddar cheese
	1 slice low fat ham
	1 slice low fat turkey
	or
v	1 cup chick peas
	3 Tablespoons honey mustard dressing
	6 saltines
	1 orange
SNACK	2 muffins
	1 cup orange juice
DINNER	1 cup Sweet and Sour Chicken*
	2 cups wild rice
	1 roll
SNACK	1 cup low fat frozen yogurt
	3/4 cup berries

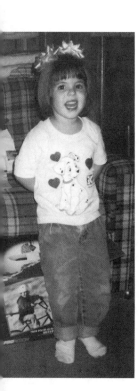

Children need models rather than critics.

– Joseph Joubert

Day 2

BREAKFAST	1 1/2 cups whole grain, unsweetened cereal 1 cup skim milk 1 banana
SNACK	1 cup low fat yogurt
LUNCH	1 Stuffed Baked Potato* 1 apple 1 kiwi fruit
SNACK	1/2 cup low fat dressing* for dipping raw carrot or celery sticks
DINNER	2 lean beef soft tacos, make sure beef is drained and rinsed in a colander before adding seasonings or *v* 2 black bean soft tacos lettuce, tomato, reduced fat cheese, lite sour cream, and Southland Salsa* 1 cup Spanish Rice* 1 cup fat free refried beans
SNACK	1 slice angel food cake 1/2 cup strawberries 1/2 cup vanilla low fat frozen yogurt

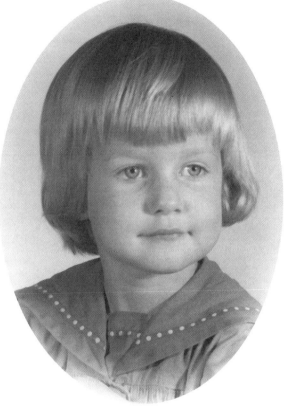

Day 3

BREAKFAST	1 bagel all-fruit jam 1 cup skim milk 1 peach
SNACK	6 graham cracker squares 1 cup low fat yogurt
LUNCH	1 turkey pita: 1 pita (whole wheat is a good choice) 2 slices fat free or low fat turkey lettuce and tomato 2 1/2 Tablespoons Cucumber Sauce*

or

v	1/2 cup garbanzo beans in place of the turkey 30 seedless grapes
SNACK	3 cups air popped popcorn (try spray-on butter flavoring) 1 cup orange juice
DINNER	1 cup meatless spaghetti sauce (try mushrooms, zucchini, other vegetables in the sauce) 1 cup pasta 1 bread sticks 1 salad with low fat dressing*
SNACK	1 cup low fat frozen yogurt 3/4 cup berries

DAY 4

BREAKFAST	1 1/2 cup whole grain, unsweetened cereal 1 cup skim milk 1 banana
SNACK	1 apple
LUNCH	Mexican salad: bed of lettuce with tomatoes and cucumbers 10 baked tortilla chips 1/2 cup reduced fat cheese 2 1/2 cup lite sour cream Southland Salsa* 1 peach
SNACK	6 graham crackers 2 Tablespoons peanut butter 1 cup orange juice
DINNER	1 square of Vegetable Lasagna 1 salad with low fat dressing* 2 slices Italian or French bread
SNACK	1 cup low fat frozen yogurt

Education is not preparation for life; education is life itself.

– John Dewey

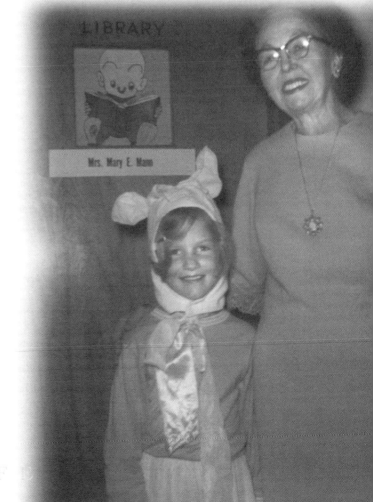

DAY 5

BREAKFAST	2 multi-grain waffles
	all-fruit jam, heated is even better!
	1 cup skim milk
	1 cup orange juice

LUNCH | 2 cups Greek Pasta Salad*

SNACK | 1 cup low fat yogurt
3/4 cup berries
3 graham cracker squares

DINNER | 3 - ounce grilled hamburger patty,
be sure to drain patty on a paper
towel before eating
1 cup Low Fat Macaroni and Cheese*
or
v 2 cups Low Fat Macaroni and Cheese*
collard greens
1 corn muffin

SNACK | 1 slice angel food cake
1/2 cup low fat frozen yogurt
1 peach

Grandchildren
are the crown of
the aged.

– Proverbs 17:6

DAY 6

BREAKFAST | 1 bagel
all-fruit jam
1 banana
1 cup skim milk

SNACK | 1 cup low fat yogurt
1 peach

LUNCH | 2 slices of cheese pizza (no meat)
any veggie toppings
1 orange

SNACK | 2/3 cup pineapple chucks

DINNER
1 fat free hot dog
1 hot dog bun
or
v 1 veggie filled pita

1 cup Slim and Thin Fries*
1 cup apple sauce, no sugar added

SNACK
1 cup low fat frozen yogurt
6 graham cracker squares

Day 7

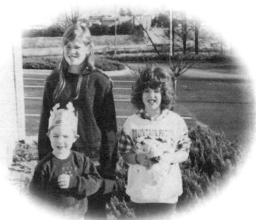

BREAKFAST
2 whole grain waffles
all-fruit jam
1 cup skim milk

SNACK
1 cup low fat yogurt
3/4 cup berries

LUNCH
2 regular tostadas from Taco Bell
1 banana

SNACK
1 cup pretzels
1/2 cup Honey Mustard, or Low Fat Ranch dresssing*
carrot sticks

DINNER
2 slices cheese pizza (no meat)
any vegetable toppings
1 salad with low fat dressing

SNACK
1 bagel
all-fruit jam
1 cup skim milk

Be sure that the all-fruit jam has no sugar added.
All the menus include vegetarian choices (*v*) , or are already a vegetarian choice.
The recipes for items marked with an asterisk (*) are included within the book.

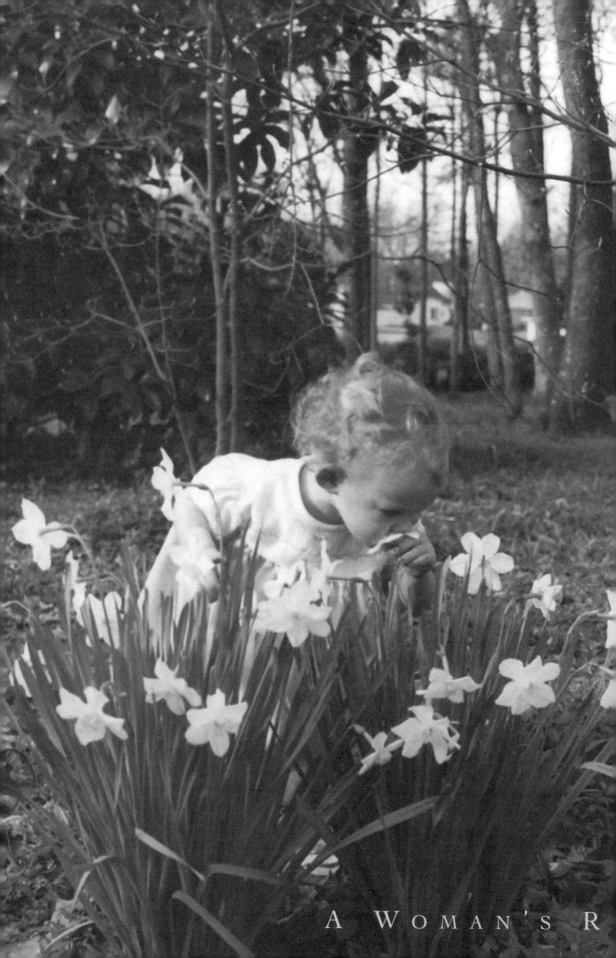

A Woman's R

BELLE'S BEST CHICKEN

4 chicken breasts, skin and all visible fat removed
4 teaspoons plain non-fat yogurt
1 cup crushed cheese crackers
1/2 cup Parmesan cheese
2 teaspoons black pepper

    Combine crackers, Parmesan cheese, and pepper.
    Coat each breast with 1 teaspoon yogurt, then roll in cracker mixture.
    Place on cookie sheet coated with non-stick spray.
    Bake at 350 degrees for 50 minutes.

Yields: 4 servings. Per serving: calories: 441; total fat: 11g; saturated fat: 4g; cholesterol: 86mg; sodium: 716mg; carbohydrates: 46g; calcium: 237mg; iron: 4mg.

GEORGIA BAKED CHICKEN

4 chicken breasts, skin and all visible fat removed
1/2 cup all-fruit peach preserves
1/2 teaspoon garlic powder
1/2 teaspoon black pepper
1 cup blush or white wine

    Preheat oven to 325 degrees.
    Arrange chicken meat side up in casserole dish sprayed with non-stick
    spray.
    Mix preserves, garlic powder, and pepper.
    Top each breast with preserves mixture.
    Pour wine over and around chicken.
    Bake for 45 minutes.

Yields: 4 servings. Calories: 332; total fat: 8g; saturated fat:2g; cholesterol: 82mg; sodium: 89mg; carbohydrates: 27g; calcium: 29mg; iron: 2mg.

CREAMY MUSTARD CHICKEN

4 boneless, skinless chicken breast halves
1/2 cup fat-free plain yogurt
3 Tablespoons Honey Mustard Dressing*
non-stick spray

Coat a non-stick skillet with non-stick spray.
Add chicken breasts and cook 4 minutes on each side (until no longer pink in center).
Remove from skillet, add yogurt and dressing to skillet.
Whisk to incorporate drippings in pan.
Add chicken and heat until heated through.

Yields: 4 servings; calories 223; total fat: 8g; saturated fat: 2g; cholesterol: 83mg; sodium:116mg; carbohydrates: 3g; calcium: 75mg, iron: 1mg.

Those who devise good meet loyalty and faithfulness.

– Proverbs 14:22

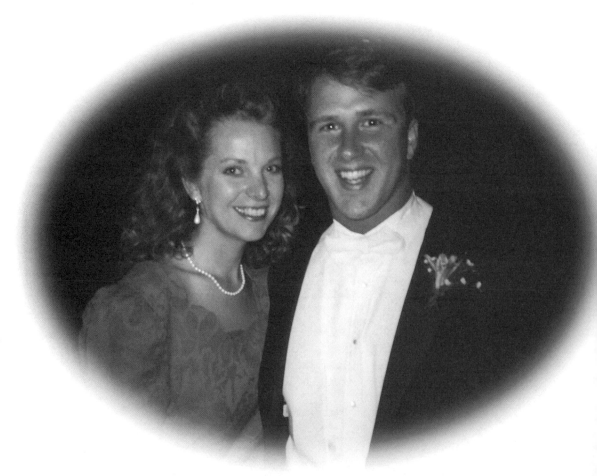

SUNDAY DINNER CHICKEN

4 to 6 chicken breasts, all skin and visible fat removed
2 onions, sliced into rings
8 ounces sliced mushrooms
1 teaspoon basil
2 teaspoons pepper
2 cups white or blush wine

Place chicken in large casserole sprayed with Pam.
Place onion and mushrooms around chicken.
Sprinkle with basil and pepper.
Pour wine over and around chicken.
Cover and bake at 325 degrees for 1 1/2 hours.

Yields: 6 servings, calories: 213, total fat: 3g, saturated fat: 1g, cholesterol: 73mg; sodium: 229mg, carbohydrates: 5g, calcium: 37mg, iron: 2mg.

CHICKEN CHABLIS PUFFS

4 boneless, skinless chicken breasts
   non-stick vegetable spray
1 can crescent rolls
3 ounces light cream cheese, softened
1 teaspoon crushed basil
1 teaspoon garlic powder
1 can reduced-fat cream of mushroom soup
1 cup white or blush wine
1 cup sliced mushrooms
1/2 cup lite sour cream
   paprika

Sauté chicken breasts in non-stick skillet sprayed with vegetable spray.
Brown on both sides, set aside to cool.
Place two triangles of crescent dough together to make a rectangle.
Place one breast on each rectangle.
Combine cream cheese, basil, and garlic powder.
Spread cream cheese mixture onto each breast.
Wrap dough around each breast so that it is completely enclosed.
Place puffs on cookie sheet sprayed with non-stick spray.

Bake at 350 degrees for 35 minutes.

Meanwhile, combine soup, wine, and mushrooms in heavy saucepan.

Heat over medium heat for 15 minutes, stirring frequently.

Just before puffs are done, remove sauce from heat.

Whisk sour cream into sauce.

Serve each puff with about 1/2 cup sauce on top; sprinkle with paprika.

Yields: 4 servings; calories:470; total fat: 21g; saturated fat:8g; cholesterol: 105mg; sodium: 866mg, carbohydrates: 22g; calcium: 115mg; iron: 4mg.

CHICKEN STROGANOFF

4 boneless, skinless chicken breasts, cubed*

1 can fat-free chicken broth

2 onions, chopped

1 cup sliced mushrooms

1 can reduced-fat cream of mushroom soup

1 packet onion soup mix

1 cup blush wine

1 teaspoon minced garlic

1 package pasta, cooked according to package directions

1 cup lite sour cream

Sauté chicken chunks in 1/2 cup fat-free chicken broth until browned on all sides.

Add onion to chicken, and continue to sauté, adding broth as necessary. Cook for another 2 to 3 minutes.

Add sliced mushrooms and cook an additional minute.

Add cream of mushroom soup, onion soup mix, wine, garlic, and remaining chicken broth.

Cook and stir until well blended and heated through.

Remove from heat just before serving, and whisk in sour cream.

Serve over hot noodles.

* 1 pound tofu (cubed) can be substituted.

Yields: 8 10-ounce servings; calories 264; total fat: 10g; saturated fat: 4g; cholesterol: 63 mg; sodium: 501 mg; carbohydrates: 18g; calcium: 69mg; iron: 2mg.

SWEET AND SOUR CHICKEN

4   boneless, skinless chicken breast, cut into chunks
1   can fat-free chicken broth
1   Vidalia onion, sliced into 1-inch pieces
1   green pepper, sliced into 1-inch pieces
2   teaspoons minced garlic
1   large can pineapple chunks, drained; reserve liquid
2   Tablespoons brown sugar
2   Tablespoons low sodium soy sauce
    hot cooked rice

Sauté chicken in 1/2 cup of chicken broth, until browned on both sides.
Add onion, green pepper, and garlic; sauté another 3 minutes.
Combine drained pineapple juice, brown sugar, and soy sauce.
Add pineapple chunks and sauce mixture to chicken.
Cook, stirring until heated through.
Serve over rice.

Yields: 4 17-ounce servings; calories: 552; total fat: 8g; saturated fat:2 g; cholesterol: 82mg; sodium: 433 mg; carbohydrates: 79g; calcium: 53mg; iron: 4mg.

TOFU VEGETABLE STIR FRY

1/4 cup all-purpose flour
 1   teaspoon basil
1/2 teaspoon black pepper
12   ounces tofu, thinly sliced
 1   Tablespoon olive oil
 2   green pepper, sliced
 2   red peppers, sliced
 1   onion, sliced
 1   carrot, sliced
 3   Tablespoons sesame seeds

Mix together flour, basil, and pepper.
Shake in a paper bag with the tofu.
Heat the oil over medium heat in a non-stick skillet.
Add tofu, and vegetables and sauté until tofu is browned on all sides.
Sprinkle with sesame seeds.

Yields: 4 7-ounce servings; calories: 192; total fat: 11g; saturated fat: 2g; cholesterol: 0mg; sodium: 15mg; carbohydrates: 16g; calcium: 179mg; iron: 7mg.

CHICKEN ROLL-UPS

  4 boneless, skinless chicken breasts
  2 slices low fat mozzarella cheese
1/2 cup sautéed mushrooms
  1 cup bread crumbs
1/2 cup Parmesan cheese
  1 teaspoon crushed basil
  2 egg whites
  2 Tablespoons skim milk
     buttery flavored non-stick spray

Place chicken between waxed paper, and flatten with a mallet.
Place 1/2 slice of cheese and 2 Tablespoons of mushrooms on each breast.
Roll up to seal in cheese/mushrooms, then close using a wooden toothpick.
Mix egg whites and milk.
Combine bread crumbs, Parmesan cheese, and basil.
Dip each rolled breast in egg mixture, then bread crumb mixture.
Place on cookie sheet sprayed with buttery flavored vegetable spray.
Spray the tops of each roll-up with buttery spray.
Bake at 350 degrees for 45 minutes.

Yields: 8 servings; calories: 356; total fat: 11g, saturated fat 5g; cholesterol: 91mg; sodium: 619mg; carbohydrates: 21g; calcium: 365mg; iron: 3mg.

CHICKEN A LA KING

  1 green pepper, diced
  1 onion, diced
     non-stick spray
  2 cups cooked chicken chunks*
  1 can reduced-fat cream of mushroom soup
  1 can fat-free chicken broth
  1 cup white or blush wine
  1 box frozen green peas
  1 cup sliced mushrooms
  2 Tablespoons cornstarch
1/2 cup skim milk

Sauté green pepper and onion in pan sprayed with non-stick spray.
Add chicken, soup, broth, wine, green peas, and mushrooms.
Bring to slow boil over medium heat, stirring frequently.
Reduce heat and simmer for 10 minutes.
Combine cornstarch and skim milk, blend until smooth.
Add to chicken mixture to thicken.
Serve over rice, noodles, or toast.
*Cooked turkey may be used in place of the chicken.

Yields: 8 10-ounce servings; calories: 244; total fat: 8g; saturated fat: 2g; cholesterol:42mg; sodium: 452mg; carbohydrates: 17g; calcium: 57mg; iron: 2mg.

CHICKEN POT PIE

4 chicken breasts, all skin and visible fat removed
1 1-pound package frozen mixed vegetables, cooked and drained
1 can reduced-fat cream of mushroom soup
2 Tablespoons blush wine
1 small can mushrooms, drained
1 teaspoon salt
1 or more teaspoons pepper
2 cups homemade chicken broth
8 large sheets phyllo dough (found in most freezer sections)
  buttery flavored non-stick spray

Bring chicken to a boil in 10 cups of water.
Reduce heat and simmer covered for 45 minutes.
Remove chicken to cool, and refrigerate broth.
Once chicken is cooled, remove from bone and tear into bite-sized pieces.
Toss together chicken, vegetables, soup, mushrooms, wine, salt, and pepper.
Remove broth from refrigerator, discard any fat.
Add broth to chicken mixture, stir lightly until well blended.
Pour into casserole coated with non-stick spray.
Layer phyllo dough on top, spraying with buttery flavored non-stick spray between each layer.
Bake at 350 degrees for 30 to 40 minutes, or until top is browned.

Yields: 8 8-ounce servings; calories: 235; total fat: 8g, saturated fat: 2g; cholesterol: 42mg; sodium: 812mg; carbohydrates: 20g; calcium: 35mg; iron: 2mg.

CHICKEN ENCHILADAS

2 cups cooked chicken, diced
1 can diced mild green chili peppers, drained
1 onion, diced
1 cup shredded low fat Monterey Jack cheese
1 cup low fat cottage cheese
1 large can tomato sauce
1 packet enchilada sauce mix
8 corn tortillas
  non-stick spray

Combine chicken, chili peppers, onion, Monterey Jack cheese, and cottage cheese.

Mix tomato sauce and enchilada sauce until well blended.

Add 1/4 cup of enchilada sauce to chicken mixture, stir mixture until consistent.

Divide chicken mixture between the 8 tortillas.

Roll each tortilla, and place seam side down in casserole coated with non-stick spray.

Pour enchilada sauce over and around each enchilada.

Bake at 350 degrees for 30 minutes.

For cheese enchiladas, omit the chicken, and use 2 onions, and 2 cups of each of the cheeses.

Flour tortillas may be substituted for the corn tortillas.

Chicken Enchiladas Yields: 8 servings; calories: 256; total fat: 9g; saturated fat: 5g; cholesterol: 56mg; sodium: 974mg; carbohydrates: 17g; calcium: 328mg; iron: 1mg.
Cheese Enchiladas Yields: 8 servings; calories: 271; total fat: 11g; saturated fat: 8g; cholesterol: 43mg; sodium: 1030mg; carbohydrates: 16g; calcium: 590mg; iron: 0.6mg.

A child is fed with milk and praise.

– Mary Lamb

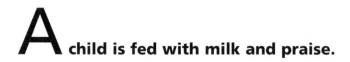

MEXICALI STEAK

1 pound round steak*, cut into thin strips
1 large onion, sliced into rings
1 green pepper, seeded and sliced into strips
1 red pepper, seeded and sliced into strips
2 teaspoons minced garlic
2 cans crushed tomatoes
2 teaspoons ground cumin
1 teaspoon salt
1 teaspoon pepper
1 beef bouillon cube
1 cup blush wine
2 Tablespoons cornstarch

Brown steak in non-stick skillet coated with non-stick spray.
Remove steak from skillet.
Add onion, peppers, and garlic, and sauté in non-stick spray.
Add steak back to mixture.
Add tomatoes, cumin, salt, pepper, and bouillon cube.
Cook over medium heat until boiling, reduce heat and simmer for 15 minutes, stirring frequently.
Combine wine and cornstarch, blend until smooth, stir into steak mixture.
Serve over Spanish rice**.

*One pound of boneless, skinless chicken breasts can be used in place of steak
**Recipe is included in book.

Yields: 8 7-ounce servings; calories: 188; total fat: 8g; saturated fat: 3g; cholesterol: 41mg; sodium: 468mg; carbohydrates: 7g; calcium: 32mg, iron: 2mg.

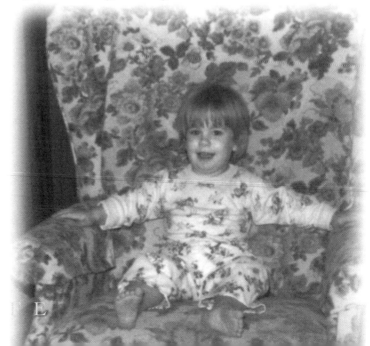

SOUTHERN ROAST

1 4- or 5-pound chuck roast, as much visible fat removed as possible
1 teaspoon minced garlic
1 Tablespoon Worcestershire sauce
1 teaspoon black pepper
2 onions, quartered
1 pound baby carrots, peeled and washed
1 cup blush wine

Place roast in casserole coated with non-stick spray.
Rub garlic onto roast.
Sprinkle Worcestershire sauce and pepper over roast.
Place onions and carrots around roast.
Pour wine over vegetables, barely sprinkling over roast.
Cover tightly with foil, and cook at 325 degrees for 2 1/2 hours.

Yields: 10 10-ounce servings; calories: 482; total fat: 17g; saturated fat: 6g; cholesterol: 206mg; sodium: 169mg; carbohydrates: 6g; calcium: 37mg; iron: 8mg.

INDIVIDUAL BEEF WELLINGTONS

8 3"x 3" filets
1 Tablespoon butter
2 cups sliced mushrooms, divided
1 cup prepared garlic/herb cheese spread
1 package pastry puff sheets (in the freezer section of most grocery stores)
   buttery flavored non-stick spray
1 can reduced-fat cream of mushroom soup
1 cup blush wine
1 cup sour cream
   fresh parsley sprigs

Brown filets on both sides in skillet sprayed with non-stick spray.
Remove filets and set aside.
Melt butter in skillet, and add 1 cup of the mushrooms.
Sauté the mushrooms in the butter for a few minutes.
Combine the mushrooms and the garlic/herb cheese, mix well.
Top each cooled filet with equal portions of the mushroom/cheese mixture.
Place each filet on a square of pastry, and top with another square of
pastry, closing on all sides.

Place wrapped filets on cookie sheet sprayed with non-stick spray.
Spray the tops of each pastry with buttery non-stick spray.
Bake at 375 degrees for 20 minutes or until pastry is browned.
Meanwhile, combine cream of mushroom soup, wine, and remaining cup of mushrooms.
Heat over medium heat until mushrooms are tender.
Remove from heat just before serving, and whisk in sour cream.
Serve mushroom sauce over each individual beef wellington.

Yields: 8 servings; calories: 376; total fat: 21g; saturated fat: 7g; cholesterol: 95mg; sodium: 543mg; carbohydrates: 13g; calcium: 81mg; iron: 4mg.

HAM AND SPINACH LASAGNA

1 cup sliced mushrooms
1 onion, chopped
1 teaspoon minced garlic
   non-stick vegetable spray
2 cup light cottage cheese
2 egg whites
1 teaspoon crushed basil
2 cups low fat mozzarella cheese
2 large cans light spaghetti sauce
1 box lasagna noodles
2 boxes frozen spinach, cooked and drained well
2 cups ham cubes*
1/2 cup Parmesan cheese

Sauté mushrooms, onion, and garlic in non-stick skillet coated with non-stick spray.
Combine mushrooms, onion, garlic, and sauce, set aside.
Combine and mix well cottage cheese, egg whites, basil, and 1 cup mozzarella cheese.
Spray a 9" x 13" pan with non-stick vegetable spray.
Spoon just enough sauce to cover bottom of pan.
Place one layer of uncooked** noodles on top of sauce.
Spoon additional sauce over noodles.
Sprinkle drained spinach evenly over sauce, then sprinkle ham chunks over spinach.
Top with another layer of noodles.
Spoon additional sauce over noodles; top with more cheese mixture.

Place final layer of noodles over cheese mixture; top with remaining sauce.
Sprinkle remaining mozzarella cheese and Parmesan cheese over top.
Bake covered at 350 degrees for 40 minutes.
Uncover and bake an additional 20 minutes.
Let cool for 10 or 15 minutes before slicing.

*2 sliced zucchini and 1 cup of baby carrots; sautéed together for a few minutes,
may be substituted for the ham chunks.
**Noodles will cook as the lasagna bakes.

Yields: 10 10-ounce servings; calories: 297; total fat: 10g; saturated fat: 4g; cholesterol: 18mg; sodium: 805mg; carbohydrates: 33g; calcium: 337mg; iron: 2mg.

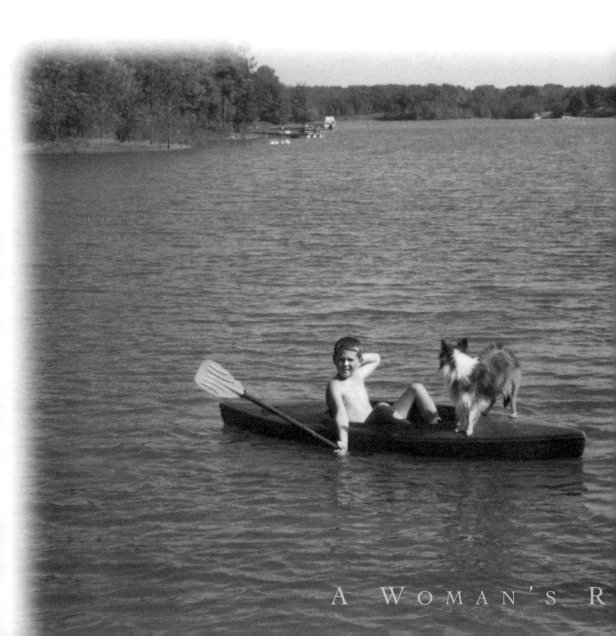

JUMBO STUFFED SHELLS

1 box jumbo shell pasta
1 zucchini, washed and sliced
1 onion, chopped
1 cup sliced mushrooms
1 teaspoon minced garlic
1 large can light spaghetti sauce
2 cup light cottage cheese
2 egg whites
1 cup shredded mozzarella cheese
1/2 cup Parmesan cheese
    non-stick vegetable spray

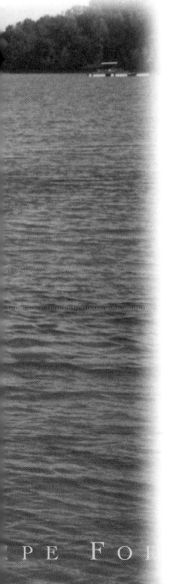

Cook pasta shells according to package
directions, drain and cool.
Sauté zucchini, onion, mushrooms, and garlic in
non-stick skillet coated with non-stick spray.
Add spaghetti sauce to sautéed vegetables.
In separate bowl, combine cottage cheese, egg
whites, and mozzarella cheese.
Spoon just enough sauce to cover bottom of
casserole coated with non-stick spray.
Fill each shell with cottage mixture, and place on
sauce in casserole.
Spoon sauce over and around stuffed shells.
Sprinkle Parmesan cheese over tops of shells.
Bake at 350 degrees for 40 minutes.

Yields: 8 10-ounce servings; calories: 248; total
fat: 9g; saturated fat: 4g; cholesterol: 15mg; sodium: 929 mg; carbohydrates: 25g; calcium:
257mg; iron: 2mg.

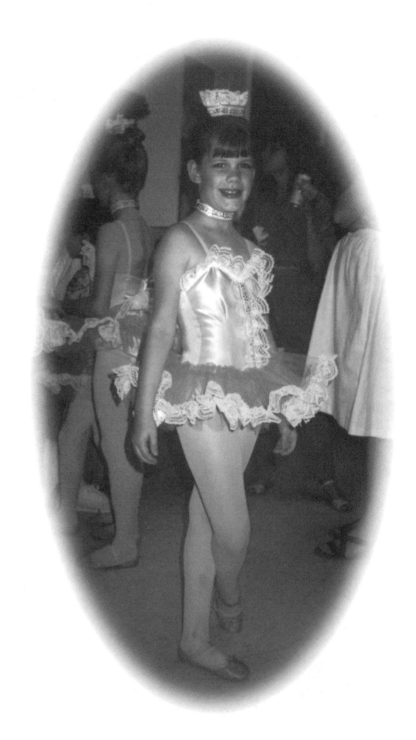

We know
that all things
work together for
good to them
that love God.

– Romans 8:28

GRILLED SEAFOOD STEAK

1 small bottle of fat-free Italian dressing
2 lemons
1/2 teaspoon tarragon
1/2 teaspoon dill weed
4 1/4- to 1/2-pound seafood steaks, such as shark, mahimahi, or salmon

Combine Italian dressing, juice from one lemon, tarragon, and dill weed.
Pour marinade into zip-type bags and add steaks.
Marinate 2 or more hours, turning every hour.
Grill for 7 minutes on each side, basting with marinade during grilling.
Serve with lemon wedges or cucumber sauce*.

*Recipe is included in the book.
Yields: 4 servings; calories: 498; total fat: 11g; saturated fat: 2g; cholesterol: 165mg; sodium; 1654mg; carbohydrates: 31g; calcium: 53mg; iron: 3mg.

LOW COUNTRY BOIL

1 pound link sausage, cut into 2" pieces
2 onions, sliced into thick rings
2 teaspoons minced garlic
2 teaspoons salt
12 medium red potatoes, scrubbed
6 ears fresh corn, shucked and cleaned
2 pounds medium to large shrimp

Fill a large soup pot with 2 gallons of water.
Add sausage, onions, garlic, and salt; bring to a boil.
Reduce heat and simmer, covered, for 10 minutes.
Add potatoes and simmer, covered over medium/low heat for 10 minutes.
Add corn and simmer, covered for 10 minutes.
Increase heat to medium.
Add shrimp, cook just a minute or two, until shrimp rises to the top and turns pink.
Serve with large salad.

Yields: 11 8-ounce serving; calories: 281; total fat: 12g; saturated fat: 4g; cholesterol: 193mg; sodium; 1084mg; carbohydrates: 16g; calcium: 59mg; iron: 4mg.

SALMON CROQUETTES

1 can salmon
1 small onion, diced and sautéed
1/8 teaspoon cayenne pepper
1 teaspoon salt
2 slices whole wheat bread, toasted and crumbled
2 egg whites
   buttery flavored non-stick spray
1 lemon

Combine salmon, onion, cayenne pepper, salt, bread crumbs, and egg whites.
Form into equal-sized patties.
Coat a non-stick skillet with buttery flavored non-stick spray.
Heat skillet on medium/high heat for 1 minute.
Add salmon, brown well on both sides.
Serve with lemon wedges.

Yields: 4 5-ounce servings; calories: 200; total fat: 8g; saturated fat: 2g; cholesterol: 41mg; sodium; 1135mg; carbohydrates: 11g; calcium: 242mg; iron: 2mg.

ORANGED PORK

6 small, boneless pork chops, all visible fat removed before cooking
3/4 cup orange marmalade
1 teaspoon garlic powder
1 cup white or blush wine

Brown chops in non-stick skillet coated with non-stick spray.
Place chops in casserole coated with non-stick spray.
Combine marmalade and garlic powder; spread evenly over chops.
Pour wine over and around chops.
Bake at 350 degrees for 30 minutes.

Yields: 6 servings; calories: 250; total fat: 5g; saturated fat: 2g; cholesterol: 52mg; sodium: 1mg; carbohydrates: 27g; calcium: 33mg; iron: 1mg.

QUICHE

2 whole eggs
8 egg whites
2 cup skim milk
1/4 teaspoon cayenne pepper
2 teaspoons salt
1 recipe filling (your choice)
1 9-inch deep-dish pie crust, unbaked
1/2 cup Parmesan cheese

Combine eggs, egg whites, milk, cayenne pepper, and salt.
Whisk until well blended.
Place filling in bottom of pie crust.
Pour egg mixture on top of filling.
Sprinkle Parmesan cheese on top.
Bake at 375 degrees for 35 to 40 minutes, or top is browned and center is firm.

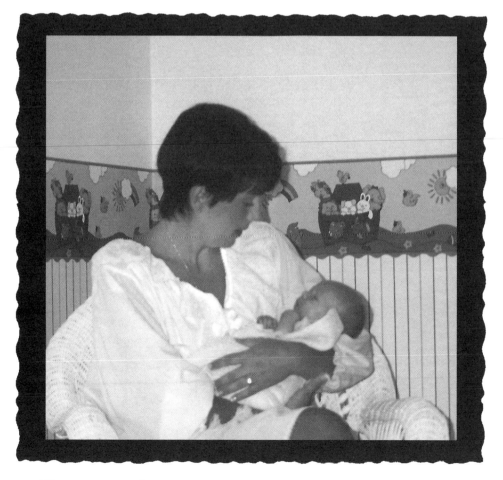

QUICHE LORRAINE

1   onion, diced
1   green pepper, diced
4   slices bacon, fried and crumbled
1/2   cup shredded Swiss cheese
1/2   cup shredded lite sharp cheddar cheese

Sauté onion and pepper in heavy skillet coated with non stick spray.
Toss together sautéed onion/pepper, bacon, and Swiss cheese.
Use according to quiche recipe.
Yields: 8 servings; calories: 186; total fat: 10g; saturated fat: 5g; cholesterol: 79mg;
sodium:939mg; carbohydrates; 7g; calcium: 365mg; iron: 0mg.

BROCCOLI AND CHEESE

1   cup fresh broccoli flowerettes, boiled for 2 minutes
1   cup shredded lite sharp cheddar cheese

Toss together, and use according to quiche recipe.
Yields: 8 servings; calories: 110; total fat: 5g; saturated fat: 3g; cholesterol: 64mg;
sodium: 758mg; carbohydrates: 5g; calcium: 213mg; iron: 0mg.

HAM, MUSHROOM, AND SWISS

1   cup ham chunks
1   cup sliced mushrooms, raw or sautéed
1   cup shredded Swiss cheese

Toss together, and use according to quiche recipe.
Yields: 8 servings; calories: 187; total fat: 10g; saturated fat: 5g; cholesterol: 88mg;
sodium: 806mg; carbohydrates: 6g; calcium: 302mg; iron: 1mg.

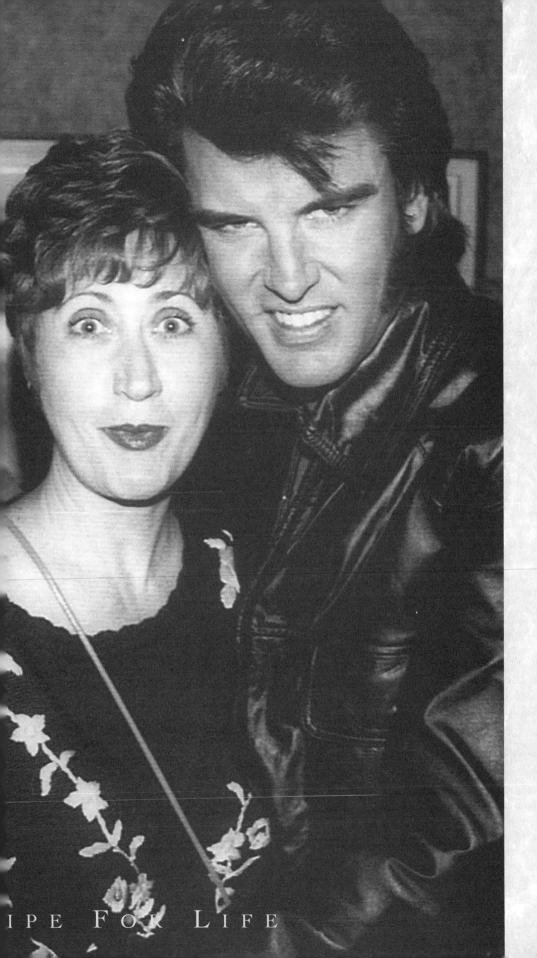

FILLINGS

Low Fat Macaroni and Cheese

1 8-ounce box macaroni, cooked and drained
1 can evaporated skim milk
2 egg whites
1 cup shredded lite sharp cheddar cheese
1 teaspoon salt
1 teaspoon black pepper
1/2 cup fat-free Parmesan cheese

Combine cooked macaroni, evaporated milk, egg whites, salt, and pepper.
Stir until well blended.
Pour into casserole coated with non-stick spray
Sprinkle Parmesan cheese on top.
Bake at 350 degrees for 30 minutes.

Yields: 8 1/2-cup servings; calories: 244; total fat: 8g; saturated fat: 5g; cholesterol: 26mg; sodium: 546mg; carbohydrates: 25g; calcium: 439mg; iron: 1mg.

Cheese Grits

1   cup cold water
3   Tablespoons quick grits
1   teaspoon reduced calorie margarine
1/4 teaspoon black pepper
1   teaspoon salt
2   Tablespoon reduced-fat sharp cheddar cheese.

Combine cold water and grits. (Water must be cold if grits are to be smooth.)
Add margarine, pepper, and salt.
Bring to a boil. Reduce heat and cover.
Simmer for 5 minutes.
Stir in cheese until melted, serve hot.

Yields: 4 1/2-cup servings; calories: 55; total fat: 2g; saturated fat: 1g; cholesterol:
5mg; sodium: 596mg; carbohydrates: 6g; calcium: 66mg; iron: 0mg.

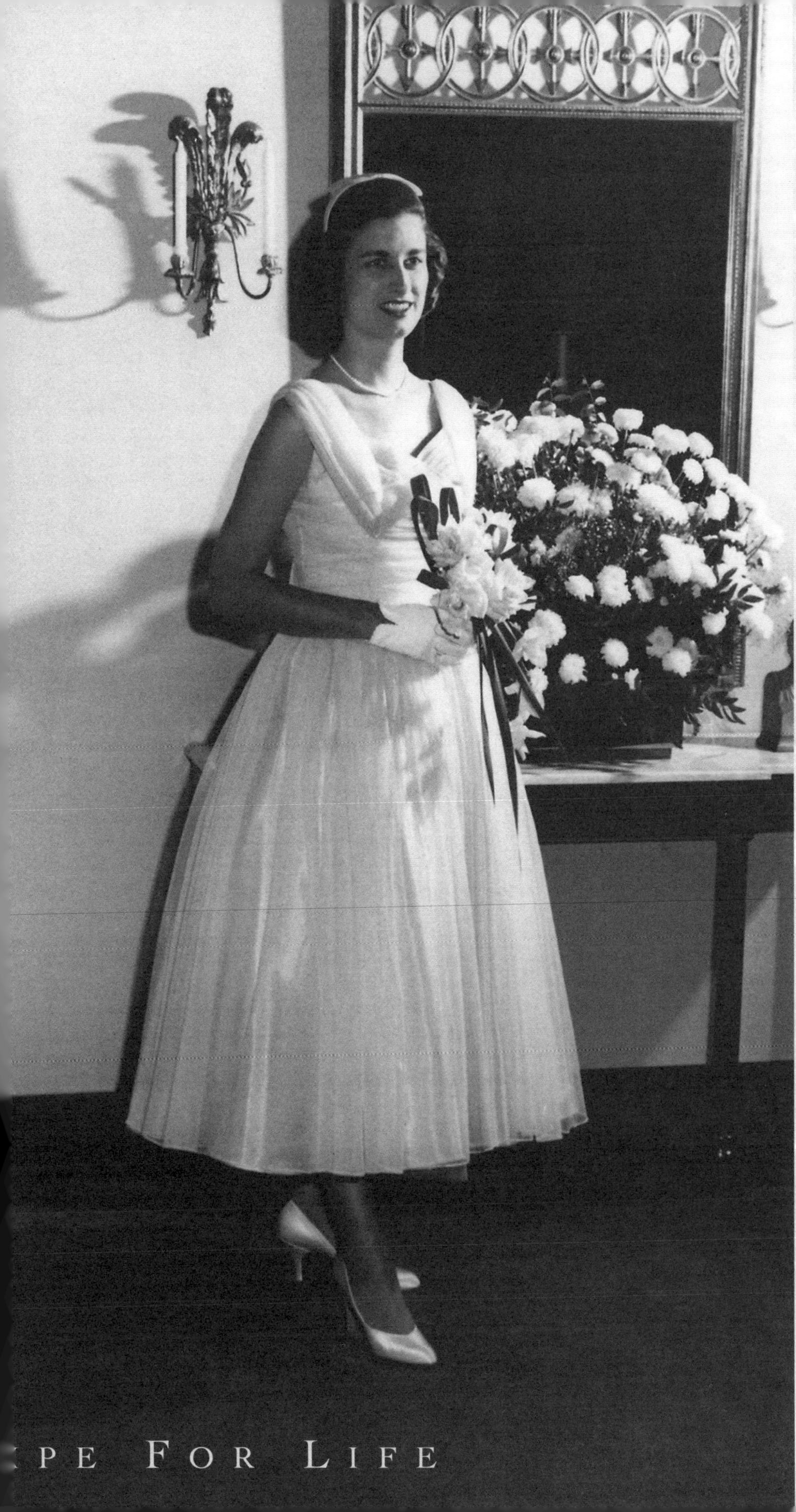

SIDE DISHES

SPANISH RICE

1 can diced tomatoes
1 cup water
1 Tablespoon reduced calorie margarine
1 teaspoon salt
1 teaspoon pepper
1 teaspoon garlic powder
1/2 teaspoon ground cumin
1 small can mild green chili peppers
1 cup long grain rice, uncooked

Combine tomatoes, water, margarine, salt, pepper, garlic powder, cumin, and green chili peppers.
Bring to a boil.
Add rice, and reduce heat to lowest stove setting.
Cook, covered on low for 20 to 25 minutes. Do not remove lid until time is up!

Yields: 6 1/2-cup servings; calories: 137; total fat: 1g; saturated fat: 0g; cholesterol: 0mg; sodium: 568mg; carbohydrates: 28g; calcium: 25mg; iron: 2mg.

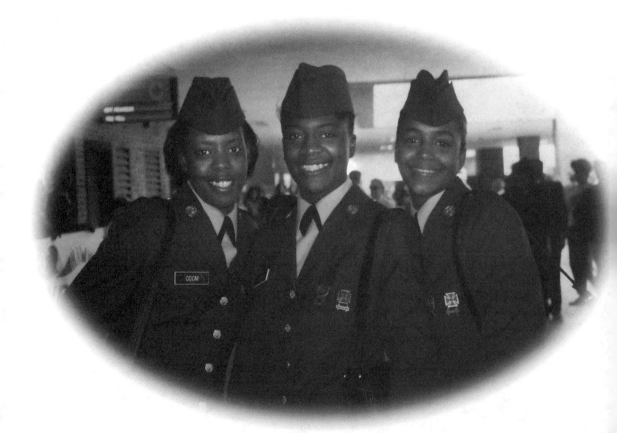

ORANGED RICE

1 cup orange juice
1 cup water
1 Tablespoon reduced calorie margarine
1 small onion, finely diced
1 teaspoon salt
1 teaspoon garlic powder
1 cup long grain rice, uncooked

Combine orange juice, water, margarine, onion, salt, and garlic powder.
Bring to a boil.
Add rice and reduce heat to the lowest stove setting.
Cover and cook on low for 20 minutes. Do not lift lid until cooking time is
up!

Yields: 6 1/2-cup servings; calories: 149; total fat: 2g; saturated fat: 0g; cholesterol:
0mg; sodium: 371mg; carbohydrates: 31g; calcium: 18mg; iron: 2mg.

SOUTHERN CAVIAR

1 1-pound package dry black-eyed peas
1 quart of water
1 teaspoon salt
2 cans fat-free chicken broth
2 cup water
1 onion, sliced into rings
1 green pepper, chopped
3 vine ripe tomatoes, chopped
1 teaspoon minced garlic
   hot sauce to taste

One can never
consent to creep when
one feels an impulse
to soar.

– *Helen Keller*

Rinse and sort peas.
Place in large pot and cover with water.
Bring to a boil, cover, and set aside for 1 hour.
Drain peas.
Combine peas, chicken broth, and 2 cups water.
Bring to a boil, reduce heat and simmer for 30 minutes.
Add remaining ingredients, and cook and additional hour.
Serve hot or cold.

Yields: 20 1/2-cup servings; calories: 86; total fat: 0g; saturated fat: 0g; cholesterol:
0mg; sodium: 158mg; carbohydrates: 15g; calcium: 29mg; iron: 2mg.

SOUTHERN CAVIAR (THE QUICK WAY)

4 cans black-eyed peas, undrained
1 can fat-free chicken broth
1 onion, sliced
1 green pepper, sliced
3 tomatoes, chopped
1 teaspoon minced garlic
  hot sauce to taste

  Combine all ingredients.
  Heat until onion and green pepper are tender.
Yields: 10 1/2-cup servings; calories: 90; total fat: 1g; saturated fat: 0g; cholesterol: 0mg; sodium: 333mg; carbohydrates: 16g; calcium: 24mg; iron: 1mg.

SUMMER SQUASH CASSEROLE

2 pounds fresh yellow summer squash, scrubbed and sliced
1 onion, sliced
1 Tablespoon reduced calorie margarine
2 teaspoons black pepper
1/2 cup evaporated skim milk
2 egg whites
1 teaspoon salt
1 cup shredded lite sharp cheddar cheese
1 cup fresh bread crumbs
1/2 cup fat-free Parmesan cheese
  buttery flavored non-stick spray

  Bring squash, onion, margarine, and 1 teaspoon pepper to a boil.
  Reduce heat and cook covered for 10 minutes, then drain.
  Combine milk, egg whites, salt, remaining 1 teaspoon of pepper, and cheese.
  Add to squash, stir to mix.
  Pour into casserole coated with non-stick spray.
  Mix bread crumbs and Parmesan cheese; sprinkle over top.
  Bake at 350 degrees for 30 minutes.
Yields: 10 1/2-cup servings; calories: 169; total fat: 7g; saturated fat: 4g; cholesterol: 21mg; sodium: 516mg; carbohydrates: 14g; calcium: 354mg; iron: 1mg.

SQUASH MEDLEY STIR FRY

2 Tablespoons reduced calorie margarine
1 cup fat-free chicken broth
1 white or yellow onion, sliced into rings
1 purple onion, sliced into rings
4 medium zucchini, sliced
6 large, fresh grown yellow summer squash, sliced
2 teaspoons black pepper
1 teaspoon salt

Melt margarine in heavy skillet over medium high heat.
Add onions (both kinds) after 1 minute.
Sauté onions for 1 minute, then add squash, salt, and pepper.
Add chicken broth as necessary, sauté for a few more minutes until desired crispness.
Yields: 9 1/2-cup servings: calories: 38; total fat: 2g; saturated fat: 0g; cholesterol: 0mg; sodium: 292mg; carbohydrates: 5g; calcium: 20mg; iron: 1mg.

STUFFED SUMMER SQUASH

1 medium onion, diced
6 medium to large summer squash, scrubbed and stem removed
1 can reduced-fat cream of celery soup
6 slices wheat bread, toasted and crumbled
1 cup shredded lite sharp cheddar cheese
1 teaspoon crushed thyme
1 teaspoon black pepper

Sauté onion in non-stick spray, until tender.
Cover squash with water in large pot.
Bring to a boil, reduce heat and cook for 3 minutes.
Drain and set aside to cool.
Combine onion, soup, bread crumbs, and spices.
Slice cooled squash in half lengthwise.
Gently scoop out inside of widest part.
Add scooped-out squash to soup mixture.
Blend well, and then stuff back equally into squash halves.
Bake at 350 degrees for 30 minutes.
Yields: 8 1/2-cup servings; calories: 182; total fat: 8g; saturated fat: 4g; cholesterol: 24mg; sodium: 626mg; carbohydrates: 17g; calcium: 307mg; iron: 2mg.

Broccoli Casserole

1	1-pound bag frozen broccoli cuts
1	can reduced-fat cream of mushroom soup
1/2	cup low cholesterol mayonnaise
2	egg whites
1	teaspoon salt
1	teaspoon pepper
1	cup shredded lite sharp cheddar cheese
1 1/2	cups crushed reduced fat cheese crackers
	buttery flavored non-stick vegetable spray

Cook and drain broccoli.
Combine cooked broccoli, soup, mayonnaise, egg whites, salt, pepper, and cheese.
Pour into casserole coated with non-stick spray.
Top with crushed crackers.
Spray top of crackers with buttery flavored spray.
Bake at 350 degrees for 30 minutes.
Yields: 12 1/2-cup servings: calories: 196; total fat: 9g; saturated fat: 4g; cholesterol: 17mg; sodium; 814mg; carbohydrates: 20g; calcium: 206mg; iron: 1mg.

Herb Vegetable Stir Fry

1	can fat-free chicken broth
1	onion, sliced into rings
1	zucchini, sliced
2	yellow squash, sliced
2	carrots, sliced into thin rounds
1	cup sliced mushrooms
1	teaspoon minced garlic
1	teaspoon crushed rosemary
1	teaspoon crushed thyme

Heat 1/2 cup chicken broth in large non-stick skillet.
Add onion and garlic; cook, stirring for 2 minutes.
Add zucchini, squash, and carrots, cooking 2 more minutes. (Use more broth if necessary.)
Add mushrooms and herbs and cook 2 more minutes.
Serve hot.

Yields: 8 1/2-cup servings; calories: 28; total fat: 0g; saturated fat: 0g; cholesterol: 0mg; sodium: 61mg; carbohydrates: 6g; calcium: 19mg; iron: 1mg.

CHEESY MASHED POTATOES

6 to 8 medium potatoes, peeled and chopped
1 Tablespoon reduced calorie margarine
1/2 cup of skim milk (or more for desired consistency)
1 teaspoon salt
1 teaspoon pepper
2 cup shredded lite sharp cheddar cheese
1/2 cup fat-free Parmesan cheese

Cover potatoes with water, and bring to a boil.
Reduce heat and cook covered for 10 minutes.
Drain and add margarine.
Mash with a potato masher.
Add milk, salt, and pepper.
Spoon into casserole sprayed with non-stick spray.
Sprinkle both cheeses evenly over top.
Bake at 350 degrees for 30 minutes.

Yields: 10 1/2-cup servings; calories: 243; total fat: 11g; saturated fat:7g; cholesterol: 37mg; sodium: 590mg; carbohydrates: 19g; calcium: 495mg; iron: 1mg.

SLIM AND THIN FRIES

4 medium potatoes, scrubbed, skins on
  buttery flavored non-stick spray
2 or more Tablespoons seasoned salt

Cut potatoes into strips, place on paper towels to dry.
Spray cookie sheet with non-stick spray.
Spread potatoes in a single layer.
Spray potatoes with non-stick spray; sprinkle with seasoned salt.
Bake at 425 degrees for 30 minutes, turning often with spatula.

Yields: 4 1/2-cup servings; calories: 115; total fat: 0g; saturated fat: 0g; cholesterol; 0mg; sodium: 7mg; carbohydrates: 27g; calcium: 6mg; iron: 0mg.

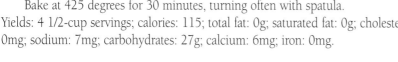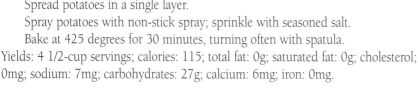

TWICE-BAKED POTATO

  1 large baking potato, scrubbed
1/2 teaspoon canola oil
  2 Tablespoons lite sour cream
  2 Tablespoons shredded lite sharp cheddar cheese
  1 Tablespoon reduced calorie margarine
     salt and pepper to taste

Coat potato with oil, and place in oven preheated to 425 degrees.
Bake for 45 minutes, check to see if done, and continue baking until potato is tender when gently squeezed.
Slice center of potato to scoop out insides, but do not cut through.
Combine potato, sour cream, cheese, margarine, salt, and pepper.
Mix well, and restuff into potato skins.
Bake at 425 degrees for 15 minutes.

Yields: 2 servings; calories: 189; total fat: 9g; saturated fat: 4g; cholesterol: 15mg; sodium: 161mg; carbohydrates: 21g; calcium: 153mg; iron: 0mg.

STUFFED BAKED POTATOES

  4 large baking potatoes, scrubbed
  2 teaspoons canola oil
  2 chicken breasts, boiled, boned and cut into chunks
  1 box frozen chopped broccoli, cooked for 2 minutes, and drained
  2 or 3 green onions, sliced
  1 Tablespoon reduced calorie margarine
  4 Tablespoons shredded lite sharp cheddar cheese
     salt and pepper to taste.

Coat each potato with 1/2 teaspoon canola oil.
Bake at 425 degrees for one hour.
Combine chicken, broccoli, onion, margarine, salt, and pepper.
Remove insides of potatoes and add to chicken mixture.
Refill the potato skins, and top each potato with 1 Tablespoon cheese.
Bake at 425 degrees for 15 minutes.

Yields: 4 servings; calories: 337; total fat: 9g; saturated fat: 3g; cholesterol: 27g; sodium: 185mg; carbohydrates: 43g; calcium: 177mg; iron: 2mg.

HEALTHY MASHED POTATOES

6 medium potatoes, peeled and quartered
1 can evaporated skim milk
   butter flavored sprinkles
   salt and pepper to taste

   Place potatoes in boiling water.
   Reduce heat and simmer on medium, covered for 10 minutes or until
   tender.
   Drain potatoes and add 2 Tablespoons buttered flavored sprinkles.
   Mash potatoes; add enough evaporated milk for desired consistency.
   Salt and pepper to taste.
Yields: 8 1/2-cup servings; calories: 110; total fat: 0g; saturated fat: 0g; cholesterol:
1mg; sodium: 41mg; carbohydrates: 23g; calcium: 97mg; iron: 0mg.

CORN PUDDING

2 boxes frozen corn, cooked for 3 minutes and drained
1 green pepper, chopped and sautéed
1 can evaporated skim milk
2 egg whites
2 slices whole wheat bread, toasted and crumbled
1 Tablespoon reduced calorie
   margarine, melted

   Combine all ingredients,
   mix well.
   Pour into casserole coated
   with non-stick spray.
   Bake at 400 degrees for 30
   minutes or until golden and
   the center is firm.
Yields: 8 1/2-cup servings; calories: 106; total fat: 2g; saturated
fat: 0g; cholesterol: 1mg; sodium:
108mg; carbohydrates: 20g;
calcium: 101mg; iron: 1mg.

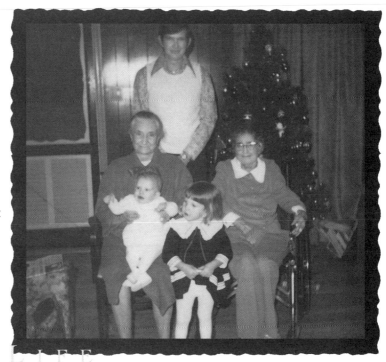

ORIENTAL MIXED VEGETABLES

1 can fat-free chicken broth
1 bunch broccoli, flowerettes cut into bite-sized pieces
1 onion, chopped
2 cups shredded cabbage
1 teaspoon minced garlic
1 can sliced water chestnuts, drained
1 can bamboo shoots, drained
2 Tablespoons soy sauce

Heat 1/2 cup chicken broth in large skillet.
Add broccoli and onion; cook for 2 minutes, stirring occasionally.
Add cabbage and minced garlic.
Cook 2 more minutes, adding more chicken broth if necessary.
Add remaining ingredients and cook an additional 2 minutes.
Yields: 6 1/2-cup servings; calories: 36; total fat: 0g; saturated fat: 0g; cholesterol: 0mg; sodium: 522mg; carbohydrates: 7g; calcium: 30mg; iron: 1mg.

The child is father of the man.

— Wordsworth

GREEN BEANS AU GRATIN

1 1-pound bag frozen green beans, cooked for 5 minutes and drained
1 Tablespoon reduced calorie margarine, melted
1 cup lite sour cream
1 cup shredded lite sharp cheddar cheese
1/2 cup evaporated skim milk
2 Tablespoons cornstarch
1 teaspoon salt
1/2 teaspoon black pepper
1/8 teaspoon cayenne pepper
1 cup fresh bread crumbs

Combine green beans, sour cream, melted margarine, and cheese; toss well.
In separate bowl, mix milk, corn stretch, salt, and peppers; blend well.
Add milk mixture to green beans; toss to coat well.
Spoon into casserole coated with non-stick spray.
Top with bread crumbs, spray with buttery flavored spray.
Bake at 350 degrees for 30 minutes.
Yields: 12 1/2-cup servings; calories: 138; total fat: 6g; saturated fat: 4g; cholesterol: 21mg; sodium: 434mg; carbohydrates: 11g; calcium: 261mg; iron: 1mg.

SNAPPY GREEN BEANS

2   cans cut green beans; one drained, one not
1   onion, sliced
2   slices bacon, fried and crumbled
1/2 cup white vinegar
1   Tablespoon sugar
2   teaspoons black pepper

    Combine all ingredients.
    Heat until heated through.

Yields: 4 1/2-cup servings; calories: 66; total fat: 2g; saturated fat: 1g; cholesterol: 3mg; sodium: 357mg; carbohydrates: 11g; calcium: 32mg; iron: 1mg.

HONEYED BABY CARROTS

1   cup whole baby carrots
1   Tablespoon honey
1   teaspoon reduced calorie margarine

    Place carrots in 1/2 cup boiling water.
    Reduce heat and simmer for 5 minutes.
    Drain carrots and add honey and margarine.
    Toss until well coated.

Yields: 2 1/2-cup servings; calories: 118; total fat: 2g; saturated fat: 0g; cholesterol: 0mg; sodium: 52mg; carbohydrates: 27g; calcium: 28mg; iron: 1mg.

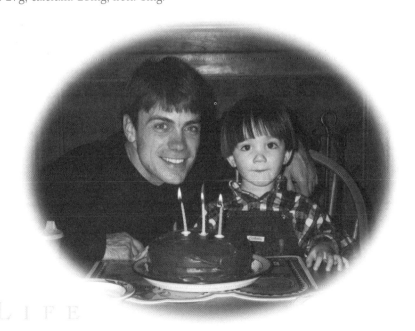

BROILED TOMATOES

4 vine ripe tomatoes
4 Tablespoons crumbled feta cheese
1/2 teaspoon basil
1/2 teaspoon crushed rosemary
1/2 teaspoon oregano

Slice tops off tomatoes.
Combine feta cheese and herbs.
Top each tomato with 1 Tablespoon feta mixture.
Bake at 325 degrees for 30 minutes.
Yields: 4 1/2-cup servings; calories: 47; total fat: 2g; saturated fat: 1g; cholesterol: 6mg; sodium: 89mg; carbohydrates: 6g; calcium: 50mg; iron: 1mg.

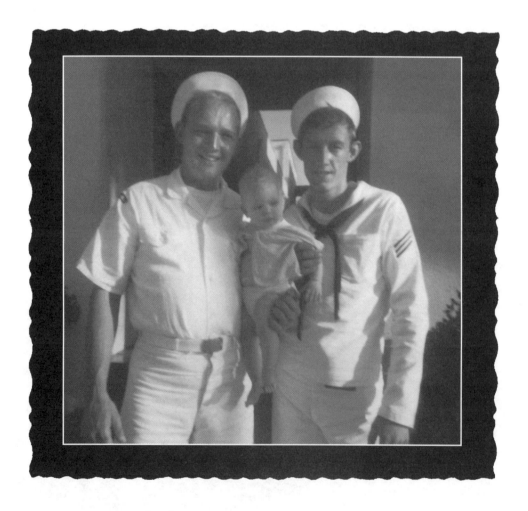

STEWED TOMATOES

4 large vine ripe tomatoes, washed well
1 teaspoon sugar
1 or more teaspoons black pepper
   hot sauce (optional)

   Place chopped tomatoes in saucepan over medium heat.
   Add remaining ingredients.
   Cook and stir for about 10 or 15 minutes.
   Serve over rice.
Yields: 4 1/2-cup servings; calories: 32; total fat: 0g; saturated fat: 0g; cholesterol:
0mg; sodium: 12mg; carbohydrates: 7g; calcium: 9mg; iron: 1mg.

LOW FAT VEGETABLES SOUTHERN STYLE

fat-free chicken broth
vegetable of your choice

To make your own fat-free chicken broth, boil some skinless, boneless chicken.
Remove chicken, and place broth in the refrigerator. Remove the fat when it rises
to the top and discard. Cook vegetables in the fat-free broth for great flavor.

HOT SPICED PEACHES

6 fresh peaches, peeled, pitted, and sliced
2 Tablespoons reduced calorie margarine, melted
2 teaspoons cinnamon
   Combine all ingredients.
   Bake at 325 degrees for 30 minutes.
Yields: 6 1/2-cup servings; calories: 61; total fat: 3g; saturated fat: 0g; cholesterol:
0mg; sodium: 24mg; carbohydrates: 10g; calcium: 15mg; iron: 0mg.

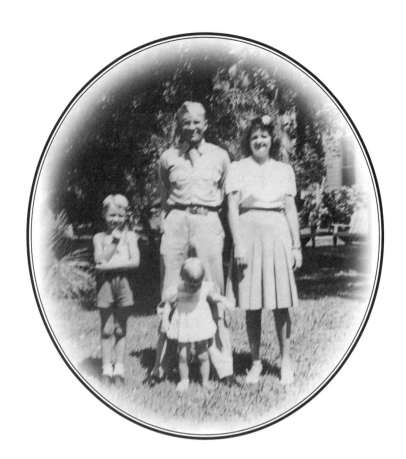

PINEAPPLE SOUFFLE

1   large can crushed pineapple, undrained
5   egg whites
1/2 cup evaporated skim milk
1/2 cup sugar
2   Tablespoons all-purpose flour
1/2 teaspoon salt
2   slices white wheat bread, cut into cubes
    buttery flavored non-stick spray

Whip together pineapple and juice, egg whites, milk, flour, and salt.
Pour into casserole coated with non-stick spray.
Place bread cubes on cookie sheet, and spray with buttery flavored spray
until all sides are coated.
Layer bread cubes on top of pineapple mixture.
Bake at 350 degrees for 30 to 40 minutes.

Yields: 8 1/2-cup servings; calories: 127; total fat: 0g; saturated fat: 0g; cholesterol:
1mg; sodium: 224mg; carbohydrates: 27g; calcium: 59mg; iron: 1mg.

SOUTHERN CORNBREAD DRESSING

5 cups crumbled cornbread
4 cups crumbled whole wheat bread toast
3 cans fat-free chicken broth
2 Tablespoons reduced calorie margarine
2 onions, chopped
2 stalks of celery, chopped
1/2 teaspoon sage
1/2 teaspoon thyme
1/2 teaspoon basil
1 teaspoon salt
1 teaspoon pepper
4 egg whites

Soak cornbread and whole wheat crumbs in 2 cans of chicken broth.
Heat margarine in non-stick skillet, and sauté onion and celery.
Mix together breads, onion/celery mixture, seasonings, and egg whites.
Toss well, then add remaining chicken broth.
Bake uncovered at 400 degrees for 45 minutes.
Yields: 12 1-cup servings; calories: 405; total fat: 10g; saturated fat: 2g; cholesterol: 28mg; sodium: 1189mg; carbohydrates: 68g; calcium: 240mg; iron: 5mg.

POTATO CAKES

2 cups leftover mashed potatoes
2 Tablespoons reduced calorie margarine

Mold chilled potatoes into small patties.
Melt margarine in large non-stick skillet.
Brown potato patties on each side.
Yields: 4 1/2-cup servings; calories: 113;
total fat: 5g; saturated fat: 1g; cholesterol: 2mg;
sodium: 353mg; carbohydrates: 19g;
calcium: 29mg; iron; 0mg.

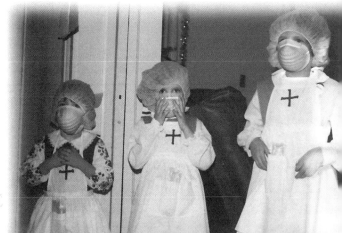

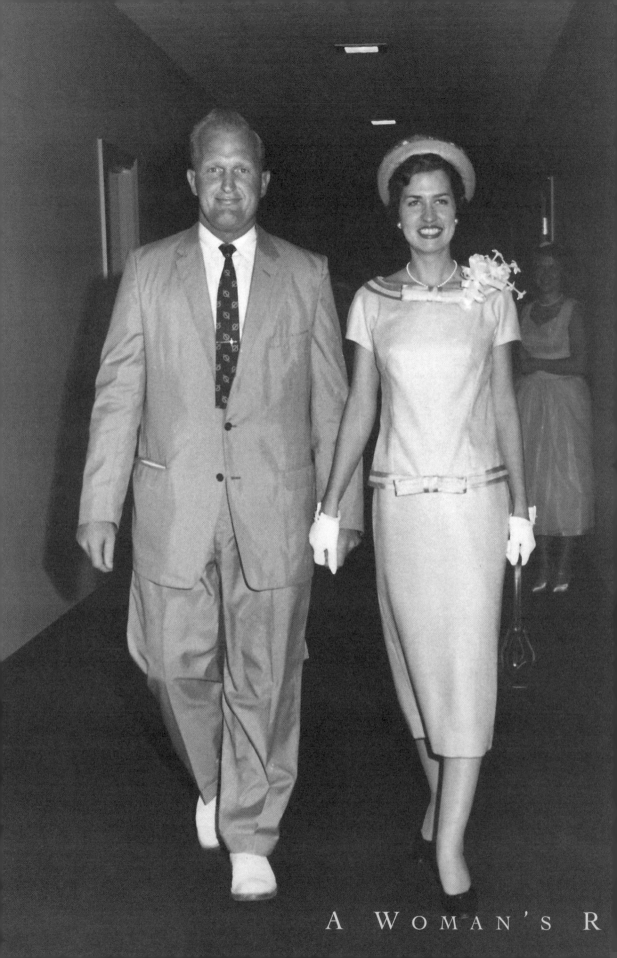

WHITE CHILI

2   boneless, skinless chicken breasts
4   cups water
1   can green chili peppers, diced
2   cans Northern white beans
2   or more teaspoons ground cumin
1   teaspoon garlic powder
1/2 teaspoon salt, or to taste
1   teaspoon white pepper
3-4 Tablespoons cornstarch
3/4 cup skim milk
1   bunch green onions, chopped

Bring the water to a boil and add chicken.
Reduce heat to medium, and boil chicken for 40 minutes.
Remove chicken from liquid and cool.
Refrigerate broth until fat rises to the top, then remove fat.
Bring broth to a slow boil.
Add chicken chunks, chili peppers, beans, cumin, garlic, salt, and pepper.
Cook over medium heat for 15 to 20 minutes.
Combine cornstarch and milk.
Slowly add cornstarch mixture to chili, and stir until thickened.
Garnish each bowl with green onions.
Yields: 8 1-cup servings. Calories per serving: 136; total fat: 1g; saturated fat: .3g;
cholesterol: 19mg; sodium: 337mg; carbohydrates: 20g; calcium: 91mg; iron: 3mg.

POLITICALLY CORRECT CHILI

4   cans fat-free chicken broth, reserve 3/4 cup
1   onion, chopped
1   green pepper, chopped
1   can Northern white beans
1   can black beans
1   can dark red kidney beans
1   can light kidney beans

1 Tablespoon ground cumin
1 teaspoon garlic powder
1 dash hot sauce
  salt to taste
2-3 Tablespoons cornstarch
  lite sour cream
  lite shredded cheddar cheese

Combine chicken broth, except 3/4 cup, onion, beans, cumin, garlic powder, hot sauce and salt.
Bring to a slow boil, reduce heat and simmer for 20 to 30 minutes.
Combine cornstarch and reserved 3/4 cup broth.
Slowly stir in cornstarch mixture, and continue stirring until thickened.
Garnish with 1 teaspoon of lite sour cream and 1 Tablespoon lite shredded cheddar cheese.

Yields: 12 3/4-cup servings. Calories per serving: 122; fat: 3.35g; saturated fat: 2g; cholesterol: 12mg; sodium: 387mg; carbohydrates: 13g; calcium: 164mg; iron: 1.76mg.

VEGETARIAN CHILI

2 cans pinto beans
2 cans kidney beans
1 large onion, chopped
1 large green pepper, chopped
2 medium cans crushed tomatoes
1 package chili seasoning mix
3 to 6 Tablespoons white corn meal
1 12-ounce bottle of non-alcoholic beer

Combine beans, onion, pepper, tomatoes, and chili seasoning mix.
Simmer uncovered for about 1 hour.
Combine corn meal and 1/2 cup water to make a paste.
Slowly add to chili to thicken.
Add non-alcoholic beer, and cook an additional 5 minutes.

Yields: 10 1-cup servings. Calories per serving: 129; fat: .73g; saturated fat: .11g; cholesterol: 0; sodium: 593mg; carbohydrates: 23g; calcium: 55mg; iron: 2mg.

TRADITIONAL VEGETABLE SOUP

2   large cans crushed tomatoes
2   cans tomato sauce
2   cans of water
1   onion, chopped
1   box frozen green beans
1   box frozen carrots
1   box frozen corn
1   box frozen baby lima beans
2   teaspoons garlic powder
1/2 teaspoon black pepper
1   teaspoon salt
1   Tablespoon Worcestershire sauce
3   Tablespoons ketchup
1   8-ounce package pasta
2   cups water

Combine tomatoes, tomato sauce, 2 cans of water, and onion.
Bring to a boil.
Add vegetables, spices, Worcestershire sauce, and ketchup.
Reduce heat and simmer for 30 minutes.
Add pasta and 2 to 4 additional cups of water.
Simmer for 8 to 10 minutes, or until pasta is done.

Yields: 12 1-cup servings. Calories per serving: 101; total fat: .43g; saturated fat: .07g; cholesterol: 0; sodium: 508mg; carbohydrates: 22g; calcium: 41mg; iron: 2mg.

BAKED POTATO SOUP

6   potatoes, scrubbed
6   teaspoons canola oil
8   cups fat-free chicken broth*
2   teaspoons salt
2   teaspoons pepper, or more if desired
1   onion, chopped and sautéed in 2 Tablespoons fat-free chicken broth
4   to 6 Tablespoons cornstarch
1   can evaporated skim milk
    lite sour cream
    shredded lite sharp cheddar cheese

Coat each scrubbed potato with 1 teaspoon oil.
Bake at 400 degrees for 1 hour. (Do not wrap in foil.)
Remove potatoes from oven, and let cool.
Bring chicken broth to a boil, then add salt, pepper, and onion.
Chop potatoes into bite-sized pieces.
Add potatoes to broth, and simmer for 10 minutes.
Combine cornstarch and evaporated skim milk.
Slowly add to soup to thicken.
Garnish each bowl with 1 Tablespoon lite sour cream and 1 Tablespoon lite shredded sharp cheddar cheese.

Yields: 8 1-cup servings. Calories per serving: 97; total fat: 1.8g; saturated fat: .31g; cholesterol: 1mg; sodium: 777mg; carbohydrates: 16g; calcium: 83mg; iron: 1.6mg.

BLACK BEAN SOUP

2   large cans crushed tomatoes or 2 quarts fresh canned tomatoes.
2   cans black beans
1   onion, chopped and sautéed in Buttery Pam in a non-stick skillet
1/2   pound smoked turkey sausage, sliced into rounds
1   Tablespoon oregano
1/2   teaspoon black pepper
1/2   cup blush wine
     lite sour cream
1   bunch green onions, sliced

Combine all ingredients, except sour cream and green onion.
Bring to a slow boil, reduce heat.
Simmer for 20 minutes.
Garnish with 1 teaspoon lite sour cream and green onion slices.

Yields: 10 1-cup servings. Calories per serving: 123; total fat: 3.54g; saturated fat: 1g; cholesterol: 13mg; sodium: 568mg; carbohydrates: 15g; calcium: 72mg; iron: 3 mg.

Beauty, without virtue, is like a flower without perfume.

— French proverb

SUMMER SQUASH SOUP

2 pounds yellow summer squash, scrubbed
1 onion, grated
1 green pepper, seeded and diced
2 cups water
1 teaspoon white pepper
1 teaspoon salt
1 Tablespoon reduced fat margarine
2 cans fat-free chicken broth
3 or 4 Tablespoons cornstarch
   lite shredded sharp cheddar cheese

Slice squash into rounds.
Place squash, onion, green pepper, and water into heavy pot.
Bring to a boil, reduce heat and cover.
Cook, covered for 10 minutes.
Mash squash. (Do not drain.)
Add white pepper, salt, margarine, and 1 can chicken broth, continue to cook over medium heat.
Combine remaining can of chicken broth and cornstarch.
Slowly add cornstarch mixture to soup to thicken, cook a few more minutes.
Garnish with 1 Tablespoon lite shredded sharp cheddar cheese.

Yields: 10 1-cup servings. Calories per serving: 88; total fat: 3.55g; saturated fat: 2g; cholesterol: 10mg; sodium: 424mg; carbohydrates: 8g; calcium: 149mg; iron: .62mg.

TOMATO BASIL SOUP

2 cans fat-free chicken broth
6 fresh tomatoes, peeled and chopped
1 Tablespoon dried basil
1 teaspoon black pepper
2 teaspoons sugar
2 Tablespoons cornstarch
1/2 cup skim milk
   fresh parsley

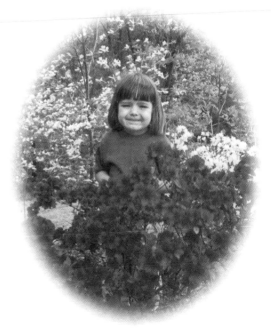

Combine chicken broth, tomatoes, basil, pepper, and sugar.
Bring to a slow boil.
Reduce heat and simmer for 10 minutes.
Combine cornstarch and milk.
Slowly add cornstarch mixture to soup to thicken.
Garnish each bowl with fresh parsley.

Yields: 10 1-cup servings. Calories per serving: 56; total fat: .56g; saturated fat: .09g; cholesterol: .25mg; sodium: 120; carbohydrates: 11g; calcium: 37mg; iron: 1mg.

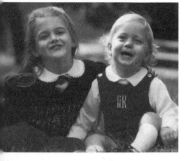

WILD BEAN SOUP

1 green pepper, chopped
1 onion, chopped
2 teaspoons minced garlic
2 cans fat-free chicken broth
2 cups cooked wild rice
1 can Northern white beans, drained
1 can black beans, drained

Sauté green pepper, onion, and garlic in 3 Tablespoons of the chicken broth.
Combine green pepper/onion mixture, chicken broth, wild rice, and beans.
Heat over medium heat until bubbly.
Simmer for 15 minutes.

Yields: 10 1-cup servings. Calories per serving: 152; total fat: .7g; saturated fat: .06g; cholesterol: 0mg; sodium: 267mg; carbohydrates: 28g; calcium: 57mg; iron: 3mg.

Give every man thine ear, but few thy voice.

– *Shakespeare*

CHINESE VEGETABLE SOUP

10 cups homemade fat-free chicken broth*
2   bunches green onions, chopped
2   boxes frozen peas and carrots
1   can sliced water chestnuts, drained
1   cup sliced mushrooms
2   cups shredded cabbage
1   Tablespoon soy sauce
2   teaspoons white pepper
4   egg whites
    chow mein noodles

Combine all ingredients except egg whites and chow mein noodles.
Bring to a boil, reduce heat and simmer, covered for 20 minutes.
Using a whisk, slowly add egg whites, whisking into the soup.
Serve immediately, topped with chow mein noodles.

Yields: 8 1-cup servings. Calories per servings: 65; total fat: 1g; saturated fat: .14; cholesterol: 0mg; sodium: 356mg; carbohydrates: 10g; calcium: 21mg; iron: 4 mg.

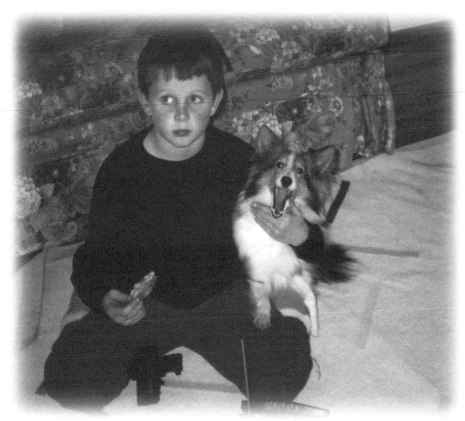

EASY SHRIMP BISQUE

2 cans tomato soup
1 can reduced fat cream of celery soup
1 can cream of shrimp soup
1 can baby shrimp, undrained
3 cups skim milk
1/2 cup blush wine
1/4 teaspoon cayenne pepper
1/2 teaspoon salt
1 lemon, sliced into rounds

Combine all ingredients, whisking until smooth.
Heat over medium low heat until heated through, do not boil.
Serve hot, garnish each bowl with a lemon curl*.

Yields: 8 1-cup servings. Calories per serving: 162; total fat: 5g; saturated fat: 2g; cholesterol: 12mg; sodium: 1297mg; carbohydrates: 21g; calcium: 143mg; iron: 2mg.

* To make a lemon curl, cut a thin slice of lemon halfway through, then twist to curl.

CRAB BISQUE

2 cans tomato soup
2 cans white crab meat, undrained
2 Tablespoons horseradish
  juice of one lemon
1 can evaporated skim milk
1 cup white or blush wine
1/8 teaspoon cayenne pepper
  fresh parsley

Combine all ingredients, and blend well.
Heat over medium heat until heated through.
Heat and stir for 6 to 8 minutes.
Serve hot and garnish with fresh parsley.

Yields: 4 3/4-cup servings. Calories per serving: 133; total fat: 2g; saturated fat: .35g; cholesterol: 31mg; sodium: 684; carbohydrates: 15g; calcium: 140mg; iron: 2mg.

BOSTON CLAM CHOWDER

    buttery flavored non-stick vegetable spray
2 cans fat-free chicken broth
1 onion, chopped
1 stalk of celery, minced
6 1-ounce rounds of Canadian bacon, minced
4 potatoes, peeled and chopped
2 Tablespoons cornstarch
2 cans evaporated skim milk
1 cup white wine
1 lemon
    fresh parsley
    salt/pepper

    Sauté onion, celery, and Canadian bacon in non-stick Dutch oven, coated
    with non-stick spray.
    Add 1/4 cup of fat-free chicken broth to onion mixture.
    Cook over medium heat for 8 minutes.
    Add clams, remaining chicken broth, and potatoes.
    Cook and stir frequently for 10 minutes.
    Combine cornstarch and 1/2 can skim milk.
    Add remaining skim milk and wine to soup.
    Slowly add cornstarch mixture.
    Cook over medium low heat until desired thickness.
    Add a lemon wedge and sprig of parsley before serving.
Yields: 12 1-cup servings. Per serving: calories: 180; total fat: 2g; saturated fat:
.60g; cholesterol: 13mg; sodium: 442mg; carbohydrates: 25g; calcium: 200mg;
iron: .80mg.

MANHATTAN CLAM CHOWDER

2   onions, chopped
6   one ounce slices Canadian bacon, chopped
2   cans crushed tomatoes
1   cup ketchup
2   cans minced clams, undrained
4   potatoes, scrubbed and chopped
2   cans fat-free chicken broth
1/8 teaspoon cayenne pepper

1 teaspoon salt
1 teaspoon pepper
2 Tablespoons corn starch
1/2 cup wine

Sauté onion and Canadian bacon in 2 Tablespoons of the fat-free chicken broth.
Cook over medium heat for 4 minutes.
Add crushed tomatoes, ketchup, clams, and clam juice.
Mix well. Add potatoes and chicken broth.
Cook and stir frequently for 10 minutes.
Add cayenne pepper, salt, and pepper.
Combine corn starch and wine, blend until smooth.
Add to soup, and stir until thickened.

Yields: 12 1-cup servings. Calories per serving: 155; total fat: 2g; saturated fat: .4g; cholesterol: 18mg; sodium: 811mg; carbohydrates: 24g; calcium: 40mg; iron: 5mg.

GAZPACHO

8 fresh tomatoes, peeled and chopped
1 cucumber, scrubbed and diced in processor
1 sweet onion, peeled and diced in processor
1 green pepper, seeded and diced in processor
2 teaspoons black pepper
2 teaspoons salt
3 teaspoons Worcestershire sauce
2 teaspoons hot sauce
2 teaspoons garlic powder
3 Tablespoons white or blush wine
   lite sour cream

Combine all ingredients and chill for several hours or overnight.
Serve in chilled bowls, topped with 1 Tablespoon lite sour cream.

Yields: 8 3/4-cup servings. Calories per serving: 65; total fat: 2g; saturated fat: 1g; cholesterol: 5mg; sodium: 577mg; carbohydrates: 10g; calcium: 40mg; iron: 1mg.

COOL STRAWBERRY SOUP

1 cup lite sour cream
1 cup fat-free plain yogurt
2 Tablespoons sugar
1 quart fresh strawberries
2 Tablespoons blush wine
   fresh mint leaves

   Combine sour cream, yogurt, sugar, and strawberries in blender.
   Blend until smooth.
   Chill for at least 24 hours.
   Serve chilled, in chilled bowls, garnished with fresh mint.

Yields: 8 1-cup servings. Per serving: calories: 115; total fat: 3g; saturated fat: 2g;
cholesterol: 11mg; sodium: 45mg; carbohydrates: 18g; calcium: 121mg; iron:
.59mg.

COOL GEORGIA PEACH SOUP

4 cups peaches, peeled and diced
1/2 cup white wine
1 cup water
2 cups apple juice
2 cinnamon sticks
1 teaspoon vanilla
   light whipped topping

   Combine peaches, wine, water, apple juice, and cinnamon.
   Bring to a boil. Reduce heat and simmer for 30 minutes.
   Remove cinnamon sticks and stir in vanilla.
   Process in small portions until smooth.
   Chill for at least 24 hours.
   Serve in chilled bowls, with a dollop of light whipped topping.

Yields: 6 1-cup servings. Per serving: calories: 111; total fat: 1g; saturated fat .4g;
cholesterol: 0mg; sodium: 5mg; carbohydrates: 24g; calcium: 33mg; iron: 1mg.

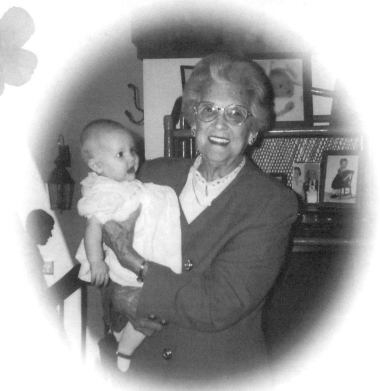

BROCCOLI AND CHEESE SOUP

3 quarts of water
2 boxes frozen, chopped broccoli
1 onion, grated
1 large block reduced fat Velvetta cheese, chunked
2 teaspoons white pepper
1 Tablespoon salt
2 teaspoons minced garlic
2 cans evaporated skim milk
4 to 6 Tablespoons cornstarch
  paprika

Bring the water to a boil.
Add broccoli and onion; simmer over medium heat for 6 minutes.
Add cheese chunks, white pepper, salt, and garlic.
Combine evaporated skim milk and cornstarch; add to soup to thicken.
Continue cooking on low heat for 15 minutes, stirring often to prevent sticking.
Garnish with paprika.

Yields: 12 3/4-cup servings. Per serving: calories: 187; total fat: 4g; saturated fat: 2.6g; cholesterol: 22mg; sodium: 1696mg; carbohydrates: 17g; calcium: 603mg; iron: 1mg.

CREAMY MUSHROOM SOUP

2 cans cream of mushroom soup *
1 16-ounce carton lite sour cream
1 small block reduced fat Velveeta cheese, chunked
1 can evaporated skim milk
1 cup blush wine
1/4 teaspoon cayenne pepper
8 ounces sliced mushrooms
  fresh parsley

Combine soups, sour cream, cheese, milk, wine, and cayenne pepper.
Whisk well until smooth.
Heat over medium heat until heated through, do not boil.
Simmer on low heat for 10 minutes.
Add sliced mushrooms.
Cook, stirring constantly until mushrooms are done.
Garnish with fresh parsley.

Yields: 8 1-cup servings. Per serving: calories:283; total fat: 17g; saturated fat: 10g;
cholesterol: 40mg; sodium: 997mg; carbohydrates: 15g; calcium: 321mg; iron: 1mg.
*Use reduced-fat cream of mushroom soup to lessen the fat content.

In youth we learn;
In age we understand.

— Marie Von Ebner-Eschenbach

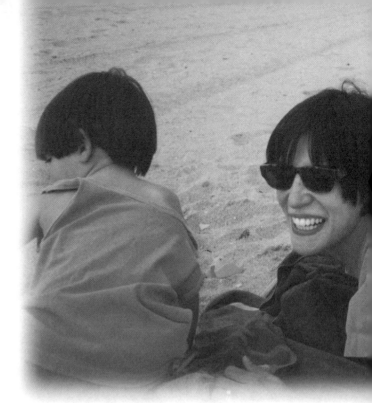

CHICKEN VEGETABLE SOUP

4 chicken breasts, skin and all visible fat removed
8 cups water
1 stalk celery
1 onion, sliced into rings
2 teaspoons salt
2 teaspoons pepper
1 teaspoon basil
1 2-pound package frozen mixed vegetables
1 8-ounce package pasta

Place chicken, water, and celery in large soup pot.
Bring to a boil, reduce heat, and simmer covered for 45 minutes.
Remove chicken to cool, remove celery and discard.
Place broth in large container in the refrigerator.
When fat has risen to the top, discard fat.
Pour broth into large soup pot.
Add chicken, onion, salt, pepper, basil, and vegetables.
Bring to a boil, then reduce heat and simmer for 20 minutes.
Add pasta, cook an additional 10 minutes.

Yields: 8 1-cup servings. Per serving: calories: 254; total fat: 2g; saturated fat: .5g; cholesterol: 36mg; sodium: 602mg; carbohydrates: 38g; calcium: 45mg; iron: 3mg.

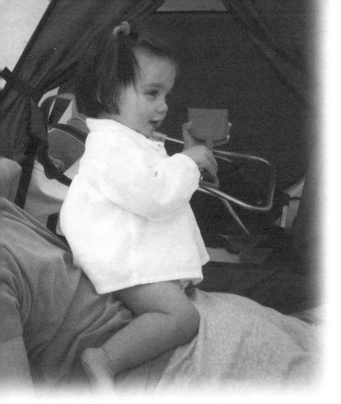

CORN CHOWDER

2   cans reduced fat cream of celery soup
1   1-pound package frozen corn
3   cans evaporated skim milk
1   green pepper, diced and sautéed in fat-free chicken broth
2   slices turkey bacon, fried crisp, drained well, and crumbled
1   teaspoon white pepper
    extra turkey bacon or paprika

   Combine all ingredients, whisking until smooth.
   Heat over medium heat.
   Reduce heat to low, simmer for 15 minutes.
   Garnish with extra crumbled bacon or paprika.

Yields: 8 1-cup servings. Per serving: calories:184; total fat: 4g; saturated fat: 1g; cholesterol: 14mg; sodium: 738mg; carbohydrates: 28g; calcium: 304mg; iron: 1mg.

It is not our exalted feelings, it is our sentiments that build the necessary home.

– Elizabeth Bowen

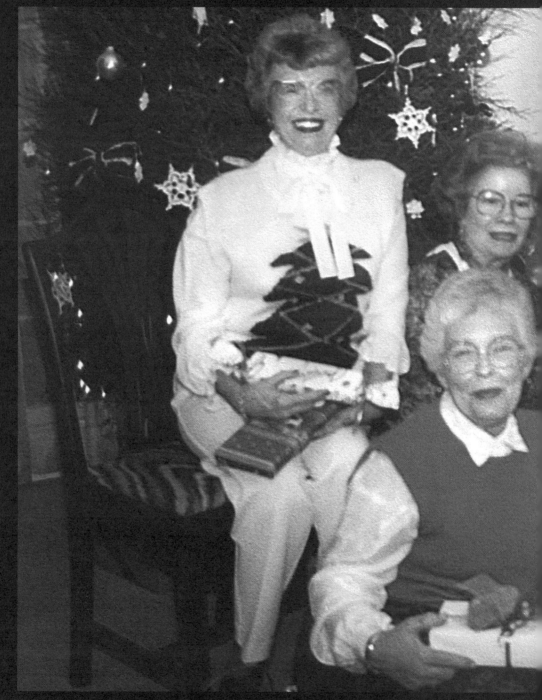

ghout

Life

Great
souls by
instinct to
each other
turn,
Demand
alliance, and
in friendship
burn.

– Addison

Stress Relief

Because stress is one of the biggest impairments to enjoying life, these next suggestions can help to alleviate some of it.

Walking is a great stress-relieving activity. A brisk walk for 20 minutes each day will help you immensely. It is acceptable to break it up into two 10-minute walks. Walking gives your body some needed activity, and you have the option to make the workout as intense or moderate as you wish. Walking is also an activity you can enjoy with a partner or your child, and you can do it indoors or out.

The following stress-busting exercises will give you some relief during your busy day:

• Place both hands behind your head. Drop your chin to your chest and hold for three seconds. Repeat several times.

• Hold both arms in front of you, palms facing outward. Slowly bring arms behind you until your shoulder blades touch. Hold for three seconds. Repeat several times.

• Place your thumbs and middle fingers together on each hand. Press the thumb and middle finger together while you slowly inhale. Hold your breath for five seconds. Slowly release your thumb and finger as you exhale. Repeat several times.

Prepare yourself for those things that tend to add unwanted stress in your life. If waiting in traffic is bothersome, take a different route, leave at a different time, or listen to CDs or tapes in your car. If waiting in line is anxiety-producing, try to run errands during times that are less busy for stores and banks.

Spend at least an hour a week on personal time. This time may be spent in an art class, learning a new cooking style, learning a foreign language, or any other activity done simply for the enjoyment. Another advantage to relishing a pleasing hobby is that it teaches children that being grown up is not all work.

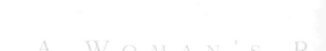

Promoting Relaxation

Families today are bombarded with activities. Although many activities are fun, such active lifestyles can lead to stress. Here are some ways to help your family relax.

Value your activities by doing just one thing at a time. Eating dinner, checking homework problems, and listening to the news is just too much. Try to really enjoy a family meal together without interruptions; watch a favorite program together, which will encourage you to discuss its positive and negative aspects and how they mesh with your family's values; or simply take a walk with your partner or child.

Be sure everyone gets plenty of rest. Eliminating caffeine from your family's diet will help to promote good health, as well as good rest. Having a set bedtime will foster a better night's sleep for your children and you.

Respect each other's privacy. When I was growing up, I was never tense at the thought that I did not have a place of my own. My parents respected my privacy, and I knew that some belongings were mine alone. The right to privacy will help your child to feel more relaxed.

Maintain some family rituals in which everyone participates. Family meal time is a good start, and a family meeting is another excellent choice. When everyone feels they are really a significant part of the group, it breeds a calmer household.

Culture opens the sense of beauty.

— Ralph Waldo Emerson

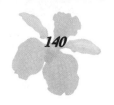

Stop Nagging

Nagging is probably one of the most time-honored ways to get our families to do what we want them to do, but it is not the most effective. In order to help get the nagging out of your home, try the following pointers.

Keep words to a minimum. Ask once, and tell what will happen if the request is ignored. For example, you ask your husband to fix the leaky faucet by a certain date; if it is not fixed, you will call a plumber. You tell your child to please pick up the toys or you will keep them in your closet for a day. Follow through; let the action take place of the begging and nagging.

Always ask nicely. A lot more can be accomplished if a please or thank you is attached.

Be realistic. A four-year old will not know exactly what to do if you simply say, "Clean up your room." Instead, give accurate directions. You may say, "I need you to pick up all of your blocks, put your dirty clothes in the hamper, and put your books on the shelf." (With younger children, give one direction at a time.)

Incorporate routines, then let the routine become the controller. Don't nag about turning off the TV for dinner time, point to the clock— "it's 6:30, time for dinner."

Have a family meeting, and seek input from everyone. Your family will be much more committed to change if they feel like they have an input.

The most important thing to do is to learn to let go! Before making a big issue out of anything, ask yourself if it is really worth it.

Time Management Skills

Learn to say "no."

Break larger tasks into smaller ones. I find this especially helpful with house-work. Working 30 minutes to one hour every evening may help to free some time on the weekends.

As you make your daily list, set priorities according to the item's importance. As you finish each item, cross it off with a colored marker—giving you a feeling of accomplishment.

Keep a list of errands that you need to run and appointments that need to be made for your family; then coordinate those that will be handled within the same trip.

Plan your week's menus ahead of time, make a grocery list, and always shop with a grocery list. This will help keep you on a budget and prevent impulse buying, and will help you to feel more organized concerning your family's mealtimes.

Delegate weekly chores to your family; include what needs to be done, as well as when it needs to be completed. Once the request is made, leave it alone.

Expect that it will get done, and then have a plan of action if it is not completed within the time frame allotted.

Whenever possible, combine two activities. For example, walking with your spouse combines needed exercise with the opportunity to discuss family and personal matters. This can prove to be a real relationship builder.

Have breakfast plans organized and items ready.

When preparing meals, always make sure that those items needing the longest cooking times are made first. Once these are underway, recipes that involve more preparation but less cooking time can be completed. By planning carefully, all foods will be ready at the same time.

Budgeting

Different stages of our lives bring distinct financial demands. Some of these demands seem more significant than others, but all must be met with thorough planning. Whether you are saving for the down payment on a house, preparing for your children's college years, building a retirement fund, meeting monthly obligations, facing a lay-off or job loss, or just getting by week to week, a financial plan must be devised.

Saving is probably the most obvious way to begin investing in your future. Even when it seems that there is nothing left to save, the commitment must be made. Take the designated savings amount out of your check first; if your company offers automatic deposit or a saving/stock program—take advantage of it. Money that is put aside before you see it will not be missed.

After discussing a budget with your partner, and looking over some financial planning books, you may want to meet with an investment counselor. You may be surprised at how little it takes to begin to strive for your short- and long-term goals. Attend the meeting as a couple, then review material as you consider the direction that will be best for your family.

SUGGESTED READINGS:

Bodar, Janet. *Kiplinger's Money-Smart Kids.* Kiplinger Books, 1993.

Eyre, Richard and Eyre, Linda. *Teaching Your Children Responsibility.* Simon & Schuster, 1984.

Godfrey, Neale and Edwards, Carolina. *Money Doesn't Grow On Trees: A Parents Guide To Raising Financially Responsible Children.* Simon & Schuster, 1994.

Hughes, Theodore and Klein, David. *The Parents' Financial Survival Guide.* Facts On File, 1995.

McCullough, Bonnie Runyan. *Bonnie's Household Budget Book.* St. Martin's Press, 1987.

Living With Teenagers

Many events that will shape the life of an adolescent occur during childhood. Building on a strong relationship will make the transition from child to adult a more positive experience. One positive approach to parenting an adolescent is to be aware that the irrational behavior, retorts, and all-knowing attitude are all signs of emerging independence. Some other suggestions include:

Adolescents and pre-adolescents need quality time with their parents. This is the only way that you will truly know your child, and this will also assure your child that you are available.

Teenagers need a parent, not just a buddy. You must continue to discipline them appropriately.

Be just as available and interested in your child's schooling as you were when he was in elementary school. Unfortunately, parental involvement in schools is reduced greatly during the middle school and high school years, when it is probably most needed.

Model good decision making techniques by including the adolescent in family decisions. This will also afford you the chance to demonstrate your family values.

If you have a disagreement with your teenager, she will win no matter what. Go into the ensuing discussions with the determination that neither of you has to lose. Be an active listener; consider your child's point of view. Respecting your teenager will promote respect from her.

Don't leave conversations just for the serious matters; enjoy talking with your adolescent. Many of your talks should occur on your child's turf, and when your child is in a relaxed mood.

SUGGESTED READINGS:

The American Academy of Pediatrics. *Caring For Your Adolescent.* Bantam Books, 1995.

Bauman, Lawrence with Riche, Robert. *The Nine Most Troublesome Teenage Problems And How To Solve Them.* Ballentine, 1986.

Caron, Ann. *Don't Stop Loving Me.* Henry Holt & Company, 1991.

Caron, Ann. *Strong Mothers, Strong Sons.* Harper Collins, 1994.

Elikind, David. *All Grown Up And No Place To Go: Teenagers In Crisis.* Addison-Wesley, 1984.

Femwick, Elizabeth, and Smith, Tony. *Adolescence.* DK Publishing, Inc., 1996.

Parrott, Les III. *Helping The Struggling Adolescent.* Aondervan Publishing House, 1993.

Shald, Jeanette; Spotts, Jules; Steinbrecher, Phyllis; and Thorpe, Douglas. *You Can Say No To Your Teenager.* Addison-Wesley Publishing Company, Inc., 1992.

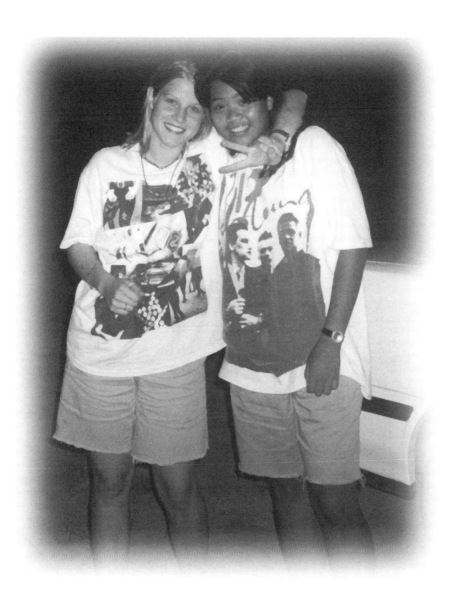

Friendship is
composed of a
single soul
inhabiting two
bodies.

– *Aristotle*

College Meal Plan Menus

During the first couple of years of college, many girls put on a few too many pounds. If you are headed off to school, and will be participating in a meal plan on campus, here is a menu plan that you may find helpful:

BREAKFAST CHOICES: 3/4 cup unsweetened cereal
1 cup skim milk
1 slice whole wheat toast,
    with all-fruit jam
1 banana or 1 cup orange juice
            or
1 bagel with all-fruit jam
1 cup skim milk or 1 cup low fat yogurt
1 banana or 1 cup orange juice

LUNCH CHOICES: 1 sandwich:
    2 slices whole wheat bread
    2 slices turkey
        or
    1/2 cup tuna
    lettuce, tomato, mustard,
    no mayonnaise
1 piece of fruit
            or
salad bar with veggies only,
no prepared salads such as potato or pasta
2 Tablespoons low calorie dressing
6 saltines
1/4 cup (one scoop) of cottage cheese
1/2 cup pineapple chunks or
        peach slices
            or
1 large baked potato with:
1 slice turkey or ham, chopped
 2 Tablespoons grated cheese
broccoli (heat stuffed potato in microwave)
1 piece of fruit

The future belongs to those who believe in the beauty of their dreams.

— Eleanor Roosevelt

DINNER CHOICES: 1 serving of meat: baked chicken breast,
                            baked fish, lean roast beef,
                            baked pork chop (make sure to
                            remove all visible fat)
                            1/2 cup rice, pasta, or potatoes
                            1 roll or other single serving
                             of bread
                            all the vegetables you want,
                            make sure they are not swimming
                            in butter or added fat
                            1 tossed salad with
                            2 Tablespoons low calorie dressing

Spaghetti with meat sauce would count as your meat and pasta choice.
2 slices of pizza with no meat toppings would count as your meat, bread, and
rice/pasta/potato choice.
2 cups of soup would count as you meat and rice/pasta/potato choice.

You may enjoy three snacks daily, preferably, one in the mid-morning, one in
the mid-afternoon, and one sometime after dinner.

SNACK CHOICES: 1 cup low fat yogurt or low fat frozen yogurt
                           1 piece of fruit
              choice of :
                           3/4 cup fat-free pretzels
                           6 vanilla wafers
                           3 graham cracker squares
                           3 cups air popped popcorn
                            (no butter)

Be sure to drink at least 8 glasses of water a day.
Exercise at least 30 minutes a day. Try walking to all of your classes.
If no amount is listed for an item, especially vegetables and salads, you may enjoy
all you want.

GREETINGS

FROM OUR HOUSE ✳

TO YOUR HOUSE ✳

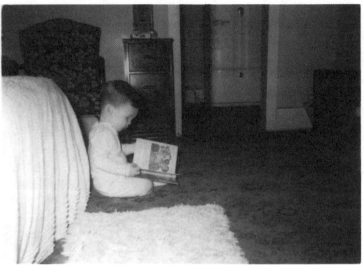

Surviving The Holiday Crunch

Remember to plan your holiday family activities so that they are age-appropriate for your children. A big meal late in the day may be fine for adults, but your little ones may not be so patient. Allowing children to eat before the scheduled meal, and then letting them watch a favorite video during the adult meal, may keep peace in the house. Your children are more likely to eat better, and the adults can enjoy a less stressful meal.

Don't be afraid to make changes in your usual holiday plans in order to incorporate your child's schedule. For younger children, try to keep them on their schedule as much as possible. Plan the extra story, caroling, gift delivery, and other supplementary activities during the good times of the day. A toddler is most secure when kept on a schedule. Try to keep bedtime as close to the usual time as possible, and remember to keep the same bedtime rituals.

Whenever possible, ask the family come to you when you have little children. Adults should able to bend a little, but it is hard to ask a small child to make a compromise, especially during such a stressful time.

Don't try to re-live your childhood through your children. Use some of your favorite memories to start some of your own family traditions, but don't try to undo some of your childhood disappointments. Know that the memories made each year will be your family's traditions.

Some of the best holiday traditions are those that happen by chance. Be open to new ways of doing things, and don't try too hard to keep the same rituals your family had when you were a child, unless they mesh well now.

The more time you spend with your children throughout the holidays, the more likely they are to cooperate when company arrives. Your child still craves your attention, so take a break from your preparations, and spend a few minutes with her so that she won't be seek attention in a negative way once your guests arrive.

Prepare your child for what is going to take place on Christmas Day. For example, if you will be leaving soon after opening the gifts, tell your child about this so she will know what to expect and will be more willing to oblige.

Do all that you can on December 23. Check to be sure you have all of the batteries you will need, and make sure that all of the unassembled gifts you have include directions.

When you go to visit relatives or in-laws, go with the attitude that you are going to have a good time. Do not allow someone else's feelings to ruin your day.

Be sure to safeguard food you will be serving for holiday meals; keep hot foods hot (140 degrees) and cold foods cold (40 degrees or colder).

If you are feeding a big crowd, buy a thermometer to check the temperatures of the food. If you are feeding a lot of people at different times, only put out a portion of the food, and then replenish as necessary. To avoid contamination, never add the new portion to a container that still has some of the older food left in it. If you are sure that the leftovers are still fresh, put in a shallow container so that they will cool quickly. Keep for four days in the refrigerator, and reheat to at least 165 degrees before serving.

If you are a guest at a party, only serve yourself from platters that you can tell are fresh. You may want to stick to safe foods such as crackers, hard cheese, or cookies.

Be sure to check toys that other family members or friends may give to your children. Watch for small parts, sharp pieces, long strings, and use your common sense.

As you shop, have a designated place to keep all receipts, so that any necessary returns will be easier. If you plan to head to the mall the day after Christmas, make a list of what you need to return, and go early so that you can find the best deals and still have the best choices. Remember that the mall will be crowded, so be prepared to be in a crowd.

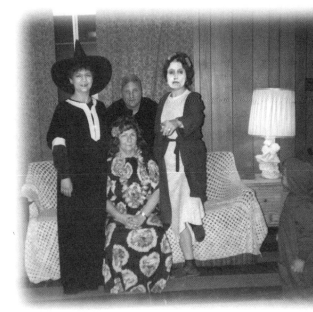

Getting Through The Holidays After The Loss Of A Family Member

There are things you can do within the family, as well as actions and words you can convey to someone who has lost a family member. Always remember that a pat on the shoulder or hug will speak volumes to a troubled friend. The following suggestions may also prove helpful.

Decide what you can handle comfortably and let your family and friends know what you can and cannot do. My family encourages others to talk about my brother, because he was and will always be such a significant part of our lives; others may feel differently.

Decide whether you can handle the responsibility of the holiday parties, a family dinner, etc., or if you need someone else to take over. Changes may be welcomed by everyone, or your family may cling to meaningful traditions.

Decide whether you will stay in town for the holidays or go to a different holiday environment.

Don't be afraid to make changes in your family routines; this can make things less painful. Open presents on Christmas Eve instead of Christmas morning; have dinner at a different time or a different place; let others take over some of the details that you have done in the past, such as delivering gifts, baking goodies, etc.

Your family may want to do something for others in memory of the person you lost:

- Give a gift in memory of the family member.
- Donate to charity the money that would have been spent on the person.
- Adopt a needy family for the holidays, or get involved in some sort of volunteer work. (In reaction to my brother's death, I sought a volunteer program to serve a Thanksgiving meal to families in my community. When I realized that there was no coordinated effort, with the help of my church and several local businesses, we began a meal that has since become a tradition of service for many families.)
- Invite a senior citizen who has nowhere else to go to enjoy the holidays with your family.

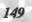

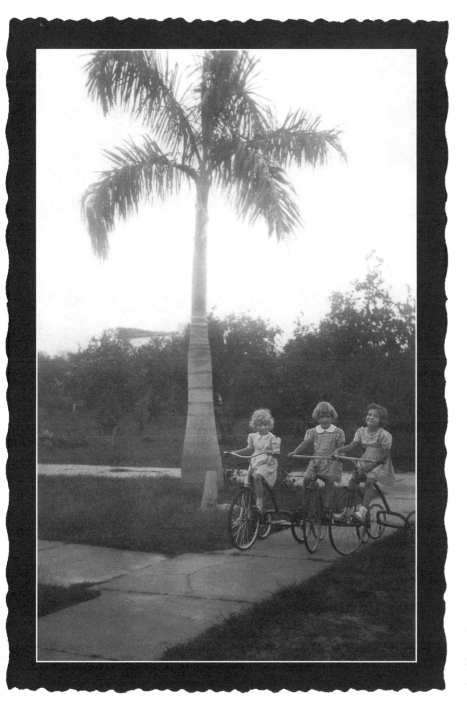

God is our
refuge and
strength, a
very present
help in trouble.

– Psalms 46:1

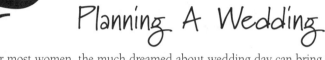

Planning A Wedding

For most women, the much dreamed about wedding day can bring about a lot of unwanted stress because this day is supposed to be perfect. One of the first obligations you have to yourself is to know that some things will be beyond your control. What you can do is plan the wedding to include those things that are meaningful to you, and be ready to react calmly to last-minute adjustments. Some considerations include:

Timing is everything! The time you choose for your wedding will have a bearing on the menu, the attire, the music, the guest list, and other aspects. Know that simplicity can be very elegant.

This is your day. Try to incorporate those ideas that were always a part of your dream wedding. Remember to be courteous in your responses to family members who have ideas that you would rather not utilize.

Keep good records of the services you will use: sign appropriate contracts with the caterer, musicians, and reception location.

Have plenty of traditional note cards ready for thank you notes. People will be very generous to you at this time, and should be thanked for time, effort, and/or gifts.

Make sure to put "you" into your selections.

This is the day which the Lord has made; let us rejoice and be glad in it.

– Psalms 118:24

SUGGESTED READINGS:

Bigel-Casher, Rita. *Bride's Guide To Emotional Survival.* Prima Publishing, 1996.

Clark, Beverly. *Planning A Wedding To Remember.* Wilshire Publications, 1995.

Gilbert, Edith. *The Complete Wedding Planner.* Warner Books, 1989.

Packham, Jo. *Wedding Ceremonies: Planning Your Special Day.* Sterling Publishing, 1993.

Post, Elizabeth L. *Emily Post's Etiquette.* Harper Collins, 1992.

In-Laws

Along with a marriage comes a new family, your in-laws, with whom you should be determined to have a quality relationship. The following tips may be helpful.

• Always do what you can to get along.

• Know that you cannot change the way someone else feels about you, but you are in control of the way that you react. Be sure that you always treat his family in a way that you would want to be treated.

- A good relationship with your in-laws will be beneficial to your relationship with your husband.
- A good relationship with your in-laws will have a positive impact on your children's lives.
- Handle all conflicts in a mature way. Be a good listener, and try to put yourself in their shoes.

SUGGESTED READINGS:
Bilofsky, Penny and Sacharow, Fredda. *Inlaws/Outlaws: How To Make Peace With His Family And Yours.* Villard Books, 1991.

Tips On Success

This is what my parents taught all of us. If you track a very successful person's life, you will see that the person made personal sacrifices, as well as worked diligently to achieve her ambition. Many times others view success as luck, but rarely is an accomplishment anything but hard work.

When planning your first career path, or even if you are changing career paths, having a sense of determination is crucial. Whether you are creating a position for yourself, or seeking a more traditional career choice, you must believe in yourself. You must have a "can do" attitude in order to achieve.

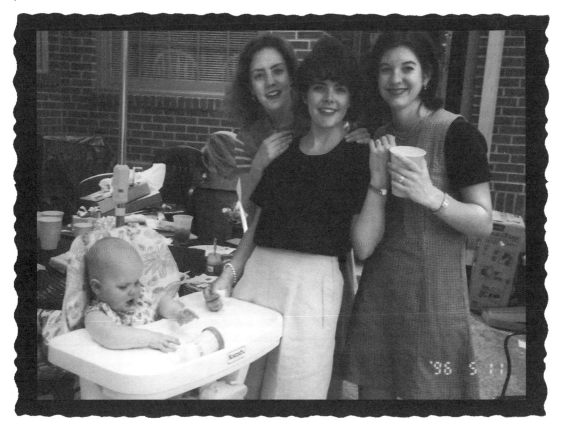

Think of something that you are good at, enjoy doing, and that someone else would pay you to do.

Seek people who are supportive.

Make a list of all the people who may have some insight into what you would like to do, or those whose ideas you respect. Make appointments for brief meetings with them, and take good notes.

Have back-up plans ready.

Make all the contacts possible—it really is who you know.

Check all parts of a new idea to make sure you are not stepping on anyone's toes. (For example, the title you choose for your new position.)

BE POSITIVE!

Read all that you can about the subject/field you have chosen. Seek any information that may be available, and use it to your advantage.

Decide on what you want, then ask for more; this will give you some room to negotiate.

Ask for what you are worth, and ask for enough that it conveys that you know your worth.

Never stop making contacts, collecting information, and always have a new idea brewing.

SUGGESTED READINGS:

Collins, Gary. *You Can Make A Difference.* Zondervan Publishing House, 1992.

Covey, Stephen. *The 7 Habits Of Highly Effective People.* Simon & Schuster, 1989.

Maxwell, John C. *Developing The Leader Within You.* Thomas Nelson Publishing, 1993.

Peale, Norman Vincent. *The Power Of Positive Living.* Fawcett-Crest, 1990.

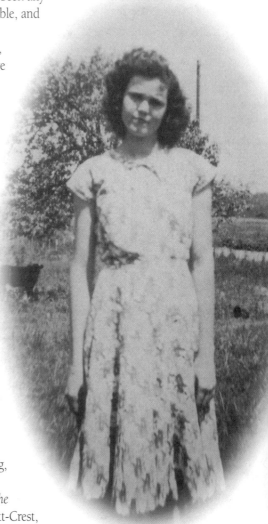

Healthy Eating Habits

We all know the importance of enjoying a healthy diet, although sometimes it is hard to stick to one because so many of the results are long range instead of immediate. In order to enjoy a healthier—and hopefully, longer—life, we must incorporate sound nutritional principles into our lifestyles.

Only bring healthy choices into your home.

Provide suitable snacks for your family.

Invest in a set of non-stick cookware.

Add an extra fruit and vegetable to your daily diet to help lower the high-fat to low-fat ratio of your regular diet.

Involve your children in the food preparation. Children are more committed to a better diet when they are involved in choosing some of the foods and preparing it.

Go vegetarian at least twice a week.

Substitute two egg whites for one egg; or evaporated skim milk in casseroles that request whole milk; and light cheeses for regular cheeses.

Don't start any habits that will have to be broken. For example, my son enjoys many vegetables, such as green peas, plain. Why add a little margarine for flavor when it isn't necessary?

Slowly make changes. Don't think of this as going on a diet, these are lifestyle changes.

Eat breakfast! This is the most important meal of the day.

Make it a rule always to say no to second servings.

Find fun things to do as a family that do not center around eating. Increase your activity level; instead of watching TV after dinner, play catch with your children.

Find hobbies that encourage activity, such as gardening, golfing, or hiking.

Always use the stairs instead of escalators or elevators.

Indulge moderately if you must splurge.

When served a large portion at a restaurant, ask for a doggie bag first, and put half the meal aside. This way you won't overeat, and you'll get to relish the wonderful food for a second meal.

Make most of your food selections from the perimeter of the grocery store; that's where you'll find the fresh fruits and vegetables, lean cuts of meats, and low fat dairy products.

Keep up-to-date on new products that are hitting the shelves. Always read the label, paying special attention to the serving size.

Differences challenge assumptions.

— Anne Wilson Schaef

Weight Loss Menu Plans (approximately 1,200 calories)

These menu plans are designed to be low fat and low cholesterol, and may encourage weight loss. In order to maintain a healthy weight loss plan, exercise must be incorporated, and as with any weight loss plan, consult your physician first.

DAY 1

BREAKFAST	1/2 bagel or 1/2 English muffin toasted with 1/4 cup reduced fat sharp cheddar cheese
SNACK	1 piece of fruit
LUNCH	1 turkey sandwich, no mayonnaise or cheese mustard/lettuce/tomato (optional) 1 piece of fruit
SNACK	30 reduced fat cheese crackers 1 piece of fruit
DINNER	1 breast, Creamy Mustard Chicken* (save one for tomorrow's lunch) 1/2 cup Corn Pudding* steamed mixed vegetables
SNACK	1 slice angel food cake 1 cup fat-free frozen yogurt

We turn not older with years, but newer every day.

– Emily Dickinson

DAY 2

BREAKFAST
3/4 cup unsweetened cereal
1 cup skim milk
1 piece of fruit

SNACK
1 piece of fruit

LUNCH
1 leftover piece of chicken
1 large salad with
2 Tablespoons low fat dressing*
6 low fat crackers

SNACK
1 piece of fruit

DINNER
1 baked, broiled, or grilled chicken
   breast (try marinated in fat-free
   Italian dressing)
1/2 cup Low Fat Macaroni and Cheese*
green beans

SNACK
1 cup fat-free frozen yogurt or
1 fat-free frozen fudge pop

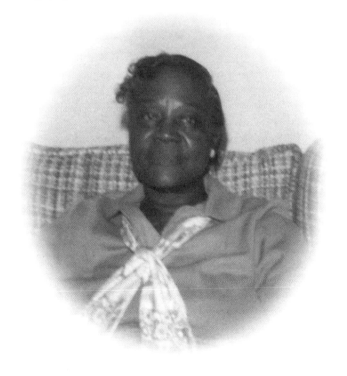

Day 3

BREAKFAST   1/2 bagel or 1/2 English muffin
                              toasted with
                          1/4 cup reduced fat sharp cheddar cheese
                          1 piece of fruit

SNACK   1 piece of fruit

LUNCH   1 Arby's regular roast beef sandwich, no mayonnaise or horseradish, (barbeque sauce is okay)
1 small salad with 1 packet of low-cal dressing

SNACK   1 piece of fruit

DINNER   1 cup Mexicali Bean Salad* on a bed of lettuce

SNACK   1 slice angel food cake
1 cup fat-free frozen yogurt

Day 4

BREAKFAST   3/4 cup unsweetened cereal
1 cup skim milk
1 piece of fruit

SNACK   1 piece of fruit

LUNCH   1 large baked potato with
1/2 cup Vegetarian chili* (canned fat-free vegetarian chili is fine)

SNACK   1 piece of fruit

DINNER   4 Jumbo Stuffed Shells*
                                 or
            1 cup pasta topped with
            1/2 cup spaghetti sauce:
                brown 1 lb. lean ground beef, rinse in
                colander, then add 1 large can
                light spaghetti sauce
            1 salad with 2 Tablespoons low fat dressing*

SNACK   1 slice angel food cake
            1 cup fat-free frozen yogurt

Day 5

BREAKFAST   1/2 bagel or English muffin toasted
                    with
            1/4 cup reduced fat sharp cheddar cheese
            1 piece of fruit

SNACK   3 graham cracker squares
            1 cup calcium-added orange juice

LUNCH   1 grilled chicken sandwich, no
                mayonnaise, and unbuttered bun
            1 small side salad with 1 packet low-
                cal dressing

SNACK   1 piece of fruit

DINNER   1 square of (1/8 of the recipe) Chicken
                Pot Pie*

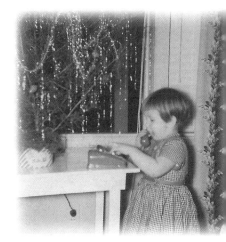

SNACK   1 waffle sprinkled with
            1 Tablespoon confectioner's sugar
           3/4 cup berries or piece of fruit

Day 6

BREAKFAST   3/4 cup unsweetened cereal
1 cup skim milk
1 piece of fruit

SNACK   3 graham cracker squares

LUNCH   1 English muffin, halved and each
topped with:
1 Tablespoon pizza sauce
2 Tablespoons low fat mozzarella
cheese
any vegetable toppings
(bake at 425 degrees until cheese
melts)
1 piece of fruit

SNACK   30 reduced fat cheese crackers

DINNER   4-ounce Grilled Seafood Steak*
1 Twice Baked Potato*
green beans or steamed broccoli

SNACK   1 slice angel food cake
1 cup fat-free frozen yogurt and
3/4 cup berries

Day 7

BREAKFAST   1 waffle with
1 Tablespoon confectioner's sugar
all-fruit jam (warmed is best)
1 cup calcium-added orange juice

SNACK   3 graham cracker squares

LUNCH   1 breast, Sunday Dinner Chicken*
1/2 cup Healthy Mashed Potatoes*
turnip greens
tomato slices
1 roll

SNACK | 1 piece of fruit

DINNER
1/2 cup scrambled Egg Beaters
1/2 cup cheese grits*
1 slice whole wheat toast
1 cup mixed fruit

SNACK
1 cup low fat frozen yogurt

Weight Maintenance Menu Plans (approximately 1,800 calories)

Day 1

BREAKFAST
1 English muffin or 1 bagel with
   all-fruit jam
1 cup skim milk
1 banana
1 cup calcium-added orange juice

SNACK
1 cup low fat yogurt
3 graham cracker squares

LUNCH
1 tuna sandwich:
   2 slices whole wheat bread
   1/2 cup Terrific Tuna Salad*
   lettuce and tomato
carrot sticks
1/2 cup pretzels

SNACK
1 cup seedless grapes

DINNER
1 cup Low Fat Macaroni and Cheese*
collard greens (exceptional source of calcium)
1 fresh sliced tomato
1 roll

SNACK
1/2 cup fat-free frozen yogurt and
1 peach

Day 2

BREAKFAST	1 1/2 cups unsweetened cereal
	1 cup skim milk
	1 piece of fruit
	1 cup calcium-added orange juice
SNACK	6 graham cracker squares
LUNCH	1 cup macaroni and cheese
	(from night before)
	1 salad with
	2 Tablespoons low fat dressing*
	1 apple
SNACK	1/4 cup low fat dressing*
	fresh vegetables for dipping
DINNER	1 breast, Belle's Best Chicken*
	1 Twice Baked Potato*
	green beans
	1 roll
SNACK	1 cup fat-free frozen yogurt
	3/4 cup berries

Day 3

BREAKFAST	1 English muffin or 1 bagel
	with all-fruit jam
	1 cup skim milk
	1 banana
	1 cup calcium-added orange juice
SNACK	1 cup low fat yogurt
LUNCH	1 Stuffed Baked Potato*
	1 salad with low fat dressing*
SNACK	1 piece of fruit
DINNER	1 cup Sweet and Sour Chicken*
	1 cup wild rice
	Honey Baby Carrots*
	1 roll

SNACK   1 banana
                        3 graham cracker squares
                        1/2 cup fat-free yogurt

Day 4

BREAKFAST   1 1/2 cups unsweetened cereal
                        1 cup skim milk
                        1 piece of fruit
                        1 cup calcium-added orange juice

SNACK   1 cup mixed fruit

LUNCH   2 cups Curried Turkey Salad*
                        on a bed of lettuce
                        2 Apple Spice Muffins*,
                           no butter/margarine

SNACK   6 graham cracker squares

DINNER   2 Cheese and Onion Enchiladas*
                        1 cup Mexican Layered Salad*

SNACK   1 cup fat-free frozen yogurt
                        3/4 cup berries

Day 5

BREAKFAST   1 English muffin or 1 bagel
                           with all-fruit jam
                        1 cup skim milk
                        1 banana
                        1 cup calcium-added orange juice

SNACK   1 cup mixed fruit

LUNCH   2 cups Mexican Layered Salad*
                        10 baked tortilla chips

SNACK   1 cup low fat yogurt
                        3/4 cup berries

Cooking is
like love. It
should be
entered into with
abandon or not
at all.

– Harriet Van Horne

DINNER	2 3-ounce Salmon Croquettes*
	1 cup cheese grits*
	1 cup cole slaw*

SNACK	6 graham crackers
	1/2 cup fat-free frozen yogurt

Day 6

BREAKFAST	1 1/2 unsweetened cereal
	1 cup skim milk
	1 piece of fruit
	1 cup calcium-added juice

SNACK	1 piece of fruit

LUNCH	1 tuna sandwich:
	2 slices light whole wheat bread
	1/2 cup Terrific Tuna Salad*
	lettuce and tomato
	cole slaw*

SNACK	1 piece of fruit

DINNER	2 cups Black Bean Soup*
	1 salad with low fat dressing*
	2 cheese drop biscuits*

SNACK	1 cup fat-free frozen yogurt
	3/4 cup berries

We arrive at the various stages of life quite as novices.

– Francois De La Rochefoucauld

DAY 7

BREAKFAST
1 English muffin or 1 bagel with all-fruit jam
1 cup skim milk
1 piece of fruit
1 cup calcium-added orange juice

SNACK
1 apple
6 saltines
1 ounce hard cheese

LUNCH
1 breast, Sunday Dinner Chicken*
1 cup Healthy Mashed Potatoes*
collards

SNACK
1 cup low fat yogurt

DINNER
3 slices Canadian bacon
2 slices multigrain waffles
3/4 cup berries
2 Tablespoons low fat whipped topping

SNACK
1 banana

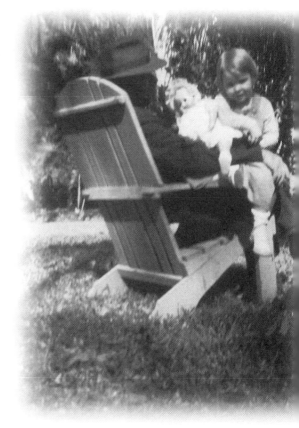

Healthy Weight Gain Menu Plan (approximately 2,500 calories)

The following menu plan will help to encourage healthy weight gain for those women who are underweight. Products such as Sustacal or Ensure can be used for the 6-ounce liquid nutrition drink. But before beginning any weight-gain plan, check with your physician first.

DAY 1

BREAKFAST	1 1/2 cups cereal 1 cup skim milk 1 banana
SNACK	1 apple 1 6-ounce can liquid nutrition drink
LUNCH	2 pieces whole wheat bread 2 slices low fat luncheon meat 1 slice cheese mustard, lettuce, tomato 1 cup calcium-added orange juice 2 small cookies
SNACK	6 graham cracker squares 1 6-ounce can liquid nutrition drink
DINNER	1 Georgia Baked Chicken* breast 1 cup wild rice green beans 1 roll
SNACK	1 cup yogurt 3/4 cup berries

DAY 2

BREAKFAST
1 cup yogurt
1 cup berries
2 bran muffins
2 teaspoons reduced calorie
margarine

SNACK
1 apple
1 6-ounce can liquid nutrition drink

LUNCH
2 slices whole wheat bread
1/2 cup Terrific Tuna Salad*
lettuce and tomato
6 vanilla wafers
1 cup skim milk

SNACK
1 orange
1 6-ounce
can liquid
nutrition
drink

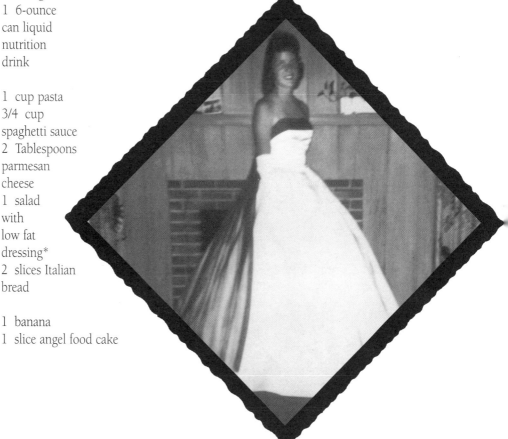

DINNER
1 cup pasta
3/4 cup
spaghetti sauce
2 Tablespoons
parmesan
cheese
1 salad
with
low fat
dressing*
2 slices Italian
bread

SNACK
1 banana
1 slice angel food cake

Day 3

BREAKFAST	1 English muffin
	2 teaspoons reduced calorie margarine
	1 egg, scrambled in Pam
	1 cup calcium-added orange juice
	1 cup skim milk
SNACK	6 graham crackers
	1 6-ounce can liquid nutrition drink
LUNCH	1 Chef's Salad:
	2 or more cups lettuce, tomato, cucumber,carrot mixture
	2 slices of cheese
	1 slice low fat luncheon meat
	low fat dressing*
	1 cup fruit cocktail
	1 roll
SNACK	1 banana
	1 6-ounce can liquid nutrition drink
DINNER	1 Bar-B-Que chicken breast
	1 cup Slim and Thin Fries*
	green beans
	2 small cubes of cornbread
SNACK	1 slice angel food cake
	1 cup low fat frozen yogurt

Luck is a matter of preparation meeting opportunity.

– Oprah Winfrey

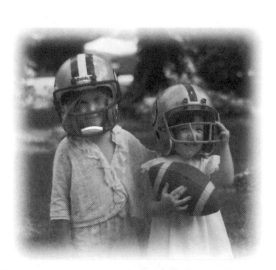

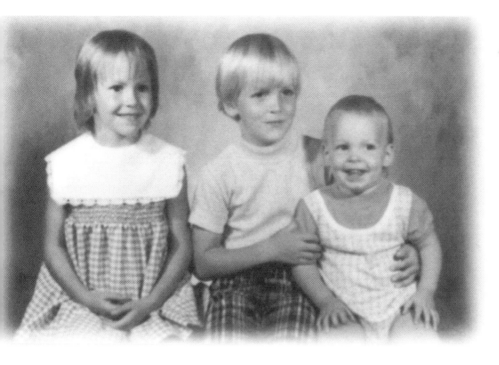

Day 4

BREAKFAST	1 1/2 cups cereal
	1 cup skim milk
	1 piece of whole wheat toast
	2 teaspoons reduced calorie margarine
	1 cup calcium-added orange juice
SNACK	1 apple
	1 6-ounce can liquid nutrition drink
LUNCH	2 bowls Chicken Vegetable Soup*
	12 saltines
	1 orange
SNACK	1 banana
	1 cup low fat frozen yogurt
DINNER	2 cups Vegetarian Chili*
	2 Tablespoons shredded cheese
	1 cube of cornbread
	1 salad with low fat dressing*
	1/2 cup pudding
SNACK	1 6-ounce can liquid nutrition drink

DAY 5

BREAKFAST	2 bran muffins
	2 teaspoons reduced calorie margarine
	1 cup skim milk
	1 banana
SNACK	1 orange
	1 6-ounce can liquid nutrition drink
LUNCH	1 single hamburger, no mayonnaise
	1 small order french fries
	1 large cookie
SNACK	1 cup peaches
	1/2 cup cottage cheese
DINNER	2 4-ounce pieces Oranged Pork Fillets*
	1 cup wild rice
	steamed broccoli
	1 cup jello with fruit
SNACK	1 6-ounce can liquid nutrition drink

DAY 6

BREAKFAST	1 1/2 cups cereal
	1 cup skim milk
	1 slice whole wheat toast
	2 teaspoons reduced calorie margarine
	1 banana
SNACK	1 orange
	1 6-ounce can liquid nutrition drink
LUNCH	2 slices whole wheat bread
	2 slices low fat luncheon meat
	1 slice cheese
	lettuce, tomato, mustard
	1 cup fruit cocktail

| SNACK | 1/2 cup low fat frozen yogurt |
| | 1/2 cup berries |

DINNER	4 ounces lean steak
	1 Twice Baked Potato*
	1 tossed salad with low fat dressing*
	1 roll

| SNACK | 1 6-ounce can liquid nutrition drink |

Day 7

BREAKFAST	1 English muffin
	2 teaspoons reduced calorie
	margarine
	all-fruit jam
	1 cup skim milk
	1 apple

| SNACK | 3 graham cracker squares |
| | 1 6-ounce can liquid nutrition drink |

LUNCH	2 slices pizza
	1 salad with low fat dressing*
	1 orange

| SNACK | 1 cup yogurt |
| | 1 banana |

DINNER	1 cup Low Fat Macaroni and Cheese*
	collard greens (very high in calcium)
	sliced tomatoes
	1 roll
	1 slice angel food cake
	1/2 cup berries

| SNACK | 1 6-ounce can liquid |
| | nutrition drink |

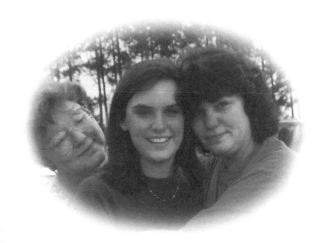

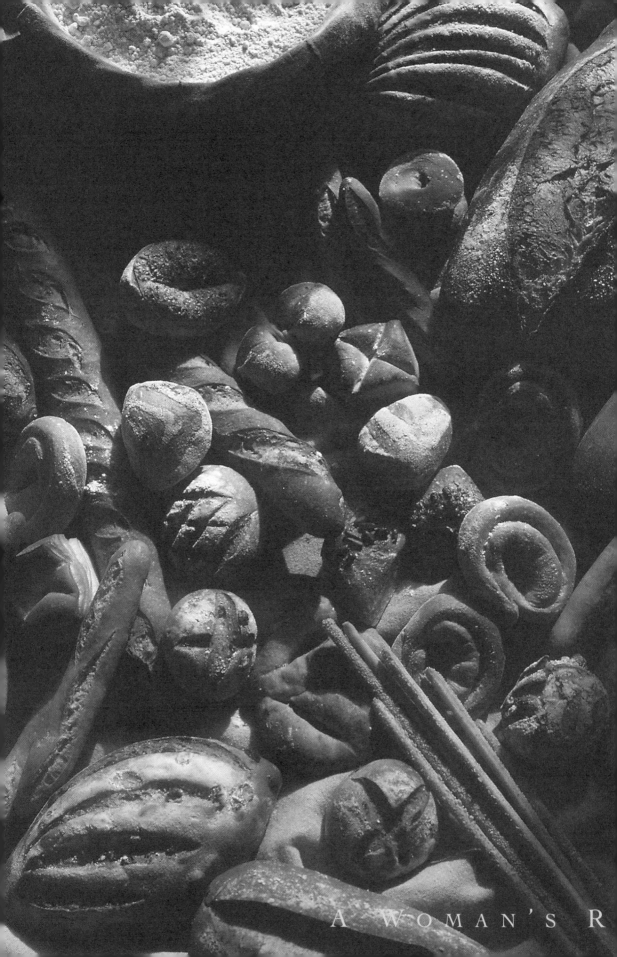

CORNBREAD

4   teaspoons canola oil
2   cups self-rising corn meal mix
1 1/4   cup skim milk
2   egg whites

Place 2 teaspoons canola oil in medium cast iron skillet.
Heat in oven at 450 degrees, while mixing cornbread.
Combine corn meal mix, milk, egg whites, and remaining 2 teaspoons of oil; mix well.
Remove skillet from oven, and spray with non-stick spray.
Pour mix into hot skillet.
Bake at 450 degrees for 18 minutes, or until golden brown.

Yields: 12 2-ounce servings; calories: 107; total fat: 2g; saturated fat: 0g; cholesterol: 0mg; sodium: 332mg; carbohydrates: 19g; calcium: 112mg; iron: 1mg.

SOUR CREAM BISCUITS

4   cups self-rising flour
1/2   cup margarine, softened
1   cup lite sour cream
1/2   cup or more skim milk

Cut margarine into flour, using two table knives.
Add sour cream and enough milk until you have a muffin batter consistency.
Spoon into muffin tins sprayed with non-stick spray.
Bake at 425 degrees for 12 minutes or until barely browned.

Yields: 20 servings; calories: 125; total fat: 4g; saturated fat: 1g; cholesterol: 2mg; sodium: 353mg; carbohydrates: 19g; calcium: 101mg; iron: 1mg.

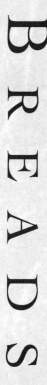

B R E A D S

HERB BISCUITS

Use preceding recipe, adding 1 to 2 teaspoons of basil, rosemary, or lemon-thyme.

CHEESE DROP BISCUITS

Use sour cream biscuit recipe, adding 1 cup of shredded lite sharp cheddar cheese. Make sure the batter is a little thicker, then drop by teaspoon or Tablespoon onto cookie sheet sprayed with non-stick spray. Bake at 450 degrees for 12 minutes.

Yields: 20 servings; calories: 157; total fat: 6g; saturated fat: 2g; cholesterol: 10mg; sodium: 442mg; carbohydrates: 19g; calcium: 203mg; iron: 1mg.

BELLE'S 60-MINUTE ROLLS

      2   cups all-purpose flour
    1/2   teaspoon salt
      2   Tablespoons sugar
      1   package yeast
      2   Tablespoons shortening
      2   Tablespoons warm water

   Dissolve yeast in 2 Tablespoons warm water.
   Sift flour, salt, and sugar together.
   Cut in shortening.
   Add dissolved yeast and warm milk.
   Work lightly until smooth.
   Roll out and cut with biscuit cutter or roll into small balls.
   Let rise 1 hour.
   Bake at 375 degrees for 20 minutes.

Yields: 12 servings; calories: 105; total fat: 2g; saturated fat: 1g; cholesterol: 0mg; sodium: 90mg; carbohydrates: 18g; calcium: 4mg; iron: 1mg.

BANANA BREAD

1/2 cup canola oil
1 1/2 cups sugar
4 egg whites
1 1/2 cups self-rising flour
1/2 cup evaporated skim milk
4 ripe bananas, mashed
1/2 cup nuts

Cream oil and sugar.
Add egg whites and mix well.
Add flour and mix well.
Add mashed bananas and nuts.
Pour batter into 2 greased and floured loaf pans.
Bake at 350 degrees for 45 minutes.

Yields: 12 4-ounce servings; calories: 314; total fat: 13g; saturated fat: 1g; cholesterol: 0mg; sodium: 230mg; carbohydrates: 48g; calcium: 89mg; iron: 1mg.

OATMEAL MUFFINS

1 cup quick cooking rolled oats
1 cup buttermilk
1/2 cup packed brown sugar
2 egg whites
1 cup self-rising flour
1/2 cup softened margarine

Soak oats in buttermilk for 30 minutes.
Add sugar, egg whites, flour, and margarine.
Pour into muffin tins coated with non-stick spray, fill 2/3 full.
Bake at 400 degrees for 25 minutes, or until browned and toothpick comes out clean.

Yields: 12 servings; calories: 140; total fat: 6g; saturated fat: 1g; cholesterol: 1mg; sodium: 212mg; carbohydrates: 19g; calcium: 70mg; iron: 1mg.

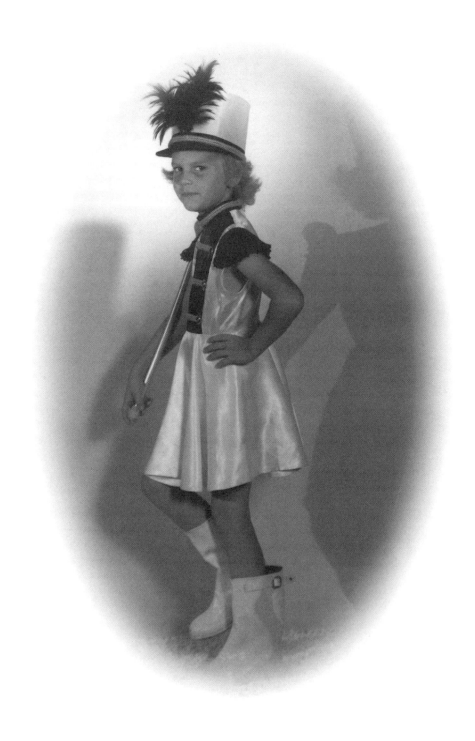

APPLE SPICE MUFFINS

1/2 cup margarine, softened
 1   cup sugar
 2   egg whites
 1   cup applesauce, no sugar added
 1   teaspoons cinnamon
 1   teaspoons ground allspice
1/2 teaspoon salt
 2   cups self-rising flour
1/2 cup almonds

Cream margarine and sugar.
Add eggs, beat well.
Add applesauce and spices.
Add flour, beat well.
Fold in nuts.
Coat miniature muffin tins with non-stick spray, fill 2/3 full.
Bake at 350 degrees for 8 to 10 minutes.

Yields: 12 servings; calories: 229; total fat: 9g; saturated fat: 1g; cholesterol: 0mg; sodium: 411mg; carbohydrates: 36g; calcium: 93 mg; iron: 1mg.

PITA CHIPS

 4 pieces of pita bread, split in half
16 teaspoons reduced calorie margarine
 4 teaspoons sesame seeds

Spread 2 teaspoons margarine on each pita round.
Sprinkle sesame seeds over all.
Bake at 350 degrees for 20 or more minutes, until crisp.

Yields: 8 servings; calories: 135; total fat: 6g; saturated fat: 1g; cholesterol: 0mg; sodium: 208mg; carbohydrates: 17g; calcium: 42mg; iron: 1mg.

What nothing earthly gives, or can destroy The soul's calm sunshine and the heartfelt joy.

– Pope

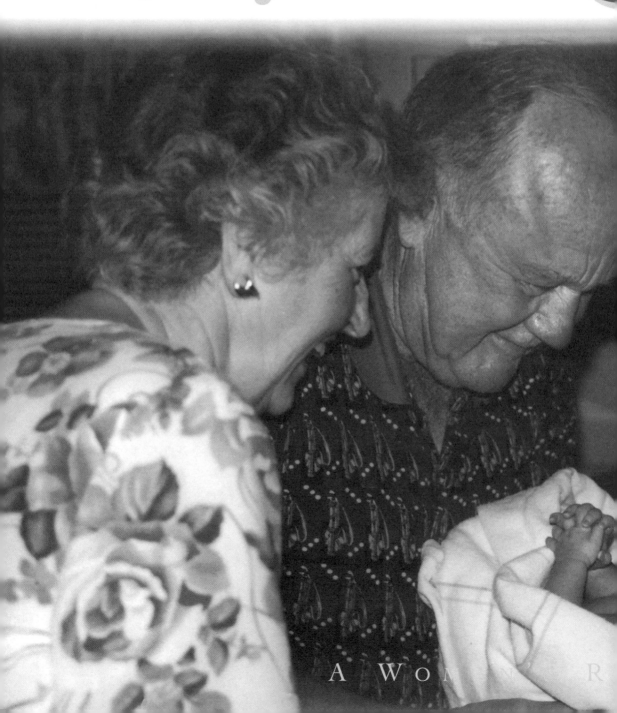

The C

A WOMAN'S R

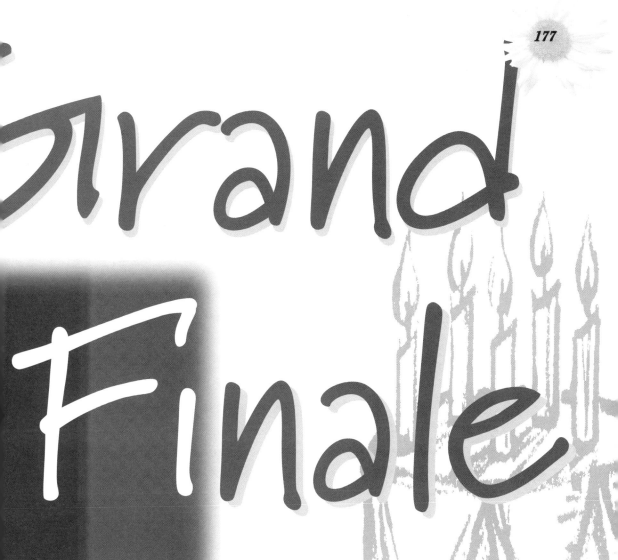

Grand Finale

Our care should not be so much to live long, as to live well.

— Seneca

Women And Cancer

Cancer—the growth of abnormal cells—is one of the most devastating illnesses a woman can face. If found early, however, the success rate of treatment greatly increases.

The American Cancer Society offers the following warning signs:
1. Unusual bleeding or discharge.
2. Thickening or lump in the breast or elsewhere.
3. Nagging cough or hoarseness.
4. Change in bowel or bladder habits.
5. Sore that does not heal.
6. Indigestion or difficulty swallowing.
7. Obvious change in a wart or mole.

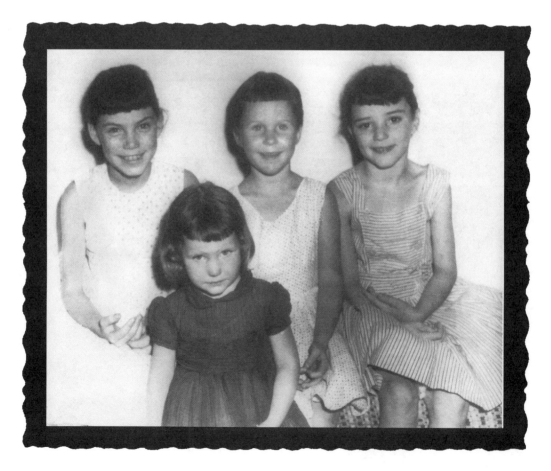

These are only warning signs, not a sure diagnosis of cancer. Nonetheless, if you have one of the warning signs, see your doctor. The following recommendations may prove helpful:

Keep updated with all advised routine care: yearly pelvic exam, yearly Pap smear, monthly breast self-exam, and yearly mammogram (if over 50 years of age). Healthy diet that is both low in fat and high in fiber.

Exercise at least 20 to 30 minutes each day.

Be aware of any changes, and call your doctor immediately if there are changes.

Watch for any changes in bleeding.

Discuss the use of estrogen with your physician.

Keep a calendar - complete with dates - if changes are noticed, when they started and how long they lasted.

If you or someone you love is diagnosed with a form of cancer, the following may prove helpful:

- Ask, ask, ask...then call back and ask some more until you are satisfied with the answers.
- Keep an ongoing list of questions.
- Talk about it. You never know who may have information that may bear on your cancer or its treatment.
- Find a support group. Your partner or children also may provide extra support.
- Continue to keep good records.
- Pray and ask for prayers.

SUGGESTED READINGS:

Komarnicky, Lydia and Rosenberg, Anne with Betancourt, Marian. *What To Do If You Get Breast Cancer*. Little, Brown, & Company, 1995.

LaTour, Kathy. *The Breast Cancer Companion*. Avon Books, 1993.

Love, Susan with Lindsey, Karen. *Dr. Susan Love's Breast Book*. Addison-Wesley, 1995.

McGinn, Kerry and Haylock, Pamela. *Women's Cancers*. Hunter House, 1993.

Runowicz, Carolyn and Haupt, Donna. *To Be Alive: A Woman's Guide To A Full Life After Cancer*. Henry Holt & Company, 1995.

Life is but a day at most.

– Burns

Hysterectomy

A hysterectomy (removal of the uterus) is one of the most common types of major surgery a woman may face. The three types of hysterectomy are:

Partial—the upper part of the uterus is removed, but the cervix remains in place.

Complete—the uterus and the cervix are removed.

Radical—the entire uterus, lymph nodes, and support structures are removed (usually the case when cancer is involved). A salpingo-oophorectomy, the removal of the ovaries and fallopian tubes, may be performed at the same time.

If you are faced with the prospect of a hysterectomy, you should first have complete confidence in your gynecologist because this assurance will help to promote a comprehensive recovery. Then, ask any questions that may arise. Once again, keep a notebook to jot down questions before your appointment or hospital work-up. Find out whether your uterus will be removed vaginally or through the abdomen. (This will be determined in the initial exam, and merited by the

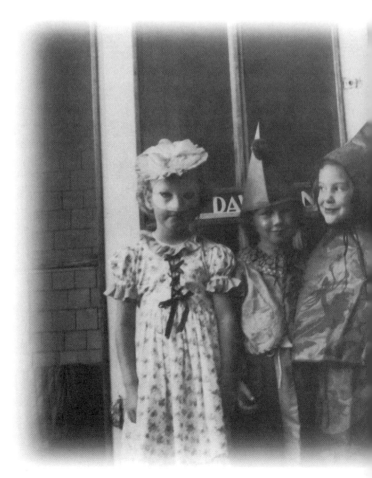

reason for surgery.) Determine a good recovery program, including your return to work as well as other activities. Explore the option of hormone replacement therapy. This will be recommended highly to treat surgical menopause.

If you have not experienced menopause, a hysterectomy will provoke it. Some of the symptoms will be even more acute, since surgical menopause occurs immediately instead of naturally over a few years. Refer to the section on menopause for guidance in understanding this phase of life.

There are many emotional considerations with a hysterectomy. Many women feel depressed with the thought of losing their womanhood. Depending on the woman's age, the fact that she can no longer become pregnant may be depressing, or it may be a relief. If you are experiencing prolonged depression, ask your gynecologist for referral to an understanding counselor.

As you begin your recovery, remember to do the following:

- Accept any help that is offered during your recovery period.
- Get plenty of rest and comply with your physician's advice.
- Seek support through a support group, or organize a group of friends or co-workers who may be going through the same thing.

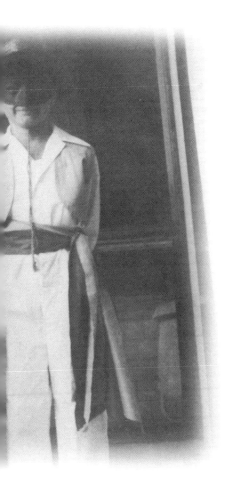

The veil which covers the face of futurity is woven by the hand of mercy.

– *Bulwer*

Menopause

There are few events in a woman's life cycle that are as potent as menopause. From hot flashes to forgetfulness, menopause is a life-changing event. The way you view menopause, how you attend to this change of life, and the support you receive, can all have an impact on you.

In the past, menopause was rarely discussed, much less studied, written about, or taken very seriously. Fortunately, today there is more information available concerning menopause. Most physicians know the variety of symptoms, as well as the diverse treatments available. There are also many books that address distinct aspects of menopause.

Unfortunately, you may have a negative view about menopause due to the observations you made of your mother's experience, as well as the negative view our society has on aging. Hopefully, both of these conditions will change. With all of the literature and support offered today to menopausal women, future generations may see this more positively.

Menopause may begin with the realization that you have missed more than one period, or you may have hot flashes or another symptom. Just as childbirth is different for each woman, menopause may include several or very few symptoms, and can be anything from brief and easy to the worst thing ever experienced.

Regardless of your symptoms, once again, you need to have that secure, supportive relationship with your gynelogist. Keep a notepad handy to jot down questions and symptoms. (Be sure to keep records of when a symptom began; this will be helpful to your health care provider.) By keeping an ongoing list, you can help to ensure that you receive answers to many of your questions. Some questions you may seek answers to include:

What information do you have on hormone replacement therapy?

Can you perform a bone density scan, or do you know where I can have a scan?

Are vision problems common during menopause?

Do you know of an active support group for menopausal women?

What information do you have on diet and its effect on me during this time?

Can you suggest a good exercise program?

SUGGESTED READINGS:

Cutler, Winnifred and Garcia, Celso-Ramon. *Menopause: A Guide For Women and Those Who Love Them.* W. W. Norton & Company, 1993.

Greer, Germaine. *The Change: Women, Aging, And Menopause.* Ballentine, 1991.

Sheehy, Gail. *The Silent Passage.* Pocket Books, 1993.

Sheehy, Gail. *New Passages.* Random House, 1995.

Menopause Menu Plan

The following is an example of a daily menu designed to provide the daily requirement of calcium through food intake. Check with your physician about your calcium requirements and on the best way to include calcium in your diet.

BREAKFAST
- 3/4 cup unsweetened cereal
- 1 cup skim milk
- 1 piece of fruit

SNACK
- 1 piece of fruit

LUNCH
- 1 large salad:
- 1 cup Romaine lettuce
- 1 boneless, skinless chicken breast, cooked and cut into chunks
- 1 cup fresh broccoli
- 1/2 cup raisins
- 2 to 3 Tablespoons low fat dressing*

SNACK
- 2 corn tortillas, warmed
- 1/2 cup Southland Salsa*

DINNER
- 1/2 cup Low Fat Macaroni and Cheese*
- 1 cup black eyed peas, cooked from dried
- 1 cup collard greens

SNACK
- 1 cup low fat frozen yogurt
- 3/4 cup berries

This combination of foods offers the recommended 1,200mg to 1,500mg of calcium. It is imperative that no substitutions be made.

Osteoporosis

Osteoporosis, a bone disease that is prevalent in women, does most damage during the menopausal years. Individuals most at risk are of Caucasian or Asian descent; have early menopause or are currently menopausal; have a family history of osteoporosis; and have low body weight and small stature.

In addition, certain lifestyles can have an impact on your chances of being affected by osteoporosis. These include: cigarette smoking, alcohol abuse, low calcium intake, vitamin D deficiency, high protein, sodium, or phosphate intake, excessive caffeine, inadequate exercise, or excessive exercise.

In order to combat osteoporosis, or its spread, you should practice the following:

Maintain regular appointments with you gynecologist.

Have a bone scan, the most progressive way to document the exact health of your bones.

Monitor calcium intake, at least 1,500 milligrams a day.

Be committed to a regular exercise program.

Practice a healthy diet.

Wrinkles should merely indicate where smiles have been.

— *Mark Twain*

Grandparents

Grandparents...just the word conjures many memories for those of us who were fortunate to have a relationship with a loving grandparent. Now that you are a parent, or if you are the grandparent, here are some pointers to consider.

The more people who love a child unconditionally, the more enriched that child's life will be.

Different generations can have diverse feelings on a variety of topics. This will grant a child the opportunity to tolerate differences of opinion.

A quality relationship with a grandparent offers the child a chance to encounter the aging process firsthand. Always answer questions honestly and simply.

Grandparents offer a connection to something that is bigger than the individual. A reliable family connection advances secure feelings within a child; children are empowered by a sense of belonging.

Family history revealed helps a child discover who he is.

When a child becomes a parent, he may feel a new bond to his parents. This will also bolster a valuable alliance among the generations.

Regardless of any former relationship hardships, the past needs to be kept in the past, and angry feelings dealt with and then put aside for the sake of the child. The beneficial attributes of the grandparent/grandchild relationship should supersede any barriers. Go into this phase of your life with the determination to get along, for the sake of the family and child.

SUGGESTED READINGS:

Ciardi, Charmaine; Orme, Cathy Nikkel; and Quatrano, Carolyn. *The Magic Of Grandparenting.* Henry Holt, 1995.

Kornhaber, Arthur. *Grandparent Power.* Crown Publishing, 1994.

Spirson, Leslie with Lehr, Claire. *The Happy Helpful Grandma* Guide. Simon & Schuster, 1994.

Caring For Aging Parents

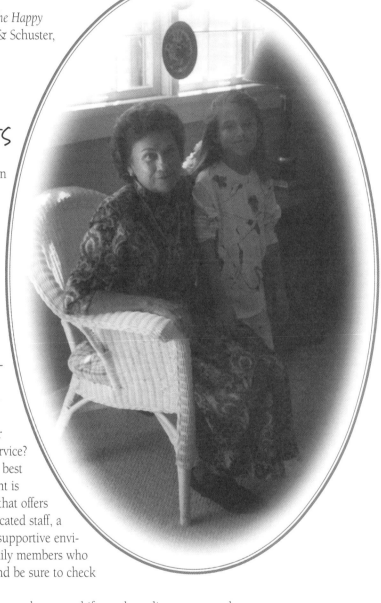

Caring for an aging parent is an immense responsibility filled with transitions and challenges. Due to the lengthened life expectancy in our society, many adults will be faced with the multiple decisions encountered when they become their parent's caregiver.

This transition will consist of hurdles for the parent, child, and the grandchildren. A conviction that things will work out is imperative for all involved, especially the adults. Considerations that need to be dealt with include:

Will the parent remain in their own home, receiving home care service?

Is a retirement home situation best for your parent? If this arrangement is necessary, choose a quality facility that offers good health care, a stable and dedicated staff, a variety of programs, and a loving, supportive environment. Ask for the names of family members who have a parent in residence there; and be sure to check references.

Will the parent be moved into your home, and if so, what adjustments need to be made within the home? Will you need the assistance of home nursing or any other form of home care for your parent?

What funds are available to help with the care of your parents, wherever they may reside?

Once a place of residence is determined, adaptations must be made within your family. If your parent continues to live at their own residence or a retirement home, plans for visiting must be made. This may be a grand opportunity for your child to strengthen his relationship with his grandparent.

If your parent will be moving into your home, some adaptations must be made. This can be a workable solution, but you will have to make a concentrated effort to encourage a smooth transition for your entire family. Some points to remember as you make the adjustment:

- Always do your best to foster your parent's dignity throughout the aging process.
- Respect your parent's privacy.
- Become an active listener. Keep the line of communication open by showing that your parent's concerns are important to you; it is vital that you simply listen to his/her needs.
- Take the opportunity to document some of your family history. Use video or audio recorder; this may be an exciting learning experience for your child. This also promotes your parent's sense of self worth, which is imperative during the aging process.
- Don't allow the care of your parent to become the only event around which your family's life revolves. Continue to plan leisure activities that you enjoy as a family, and that may or may not include your parent.

HELPFUL RESOURCES AND BOOKS

United Seniors Health Cooperative, *Long-term Care: A Dollar & Sense Guide*, and *Home Care for Older People: A Consumer's Guide*. 1331 H Street, NW, Washington, DC 2005-4706.

For free health care insurance counseling and information, The Elder Care Locator, National Association of Area Agencies on Aging, (800-677-1116).

For legal assistance dealing with aging issues, National Academy Of Elder Law Attorneys, 1604 N. Country Club Road, Tucson, AZ 85716.

Adams, Tom and Armstrong, Kathryn. *When Parents Age: What Children Can Do*. Berkley Books, 1993.

Cohen, Donna and Eisdorfer, Carl. *Seven Steps To Effective Parent Care*. G. P. Putnam's Sons, 1993.

Bland Menu Plans For The Aging (approximately 1,800 calories)

This diet was first devised for one of our physician's parents who needed very simple foods. Many times, those who are aging need more of a bland diet than that offered by a traditional menu. All items in italics are specifically for this diet, and recipes are given on pages 194-195.

Day 1

BREAKFAST	1	egg, scrambled in Pam
	1	slice whole wheat toast
	1	banana
	1	cup skim milk
SNACK	3	graham cracker squares
LUNCH	2	slices whole wheat bread
	1 to 2	slices turkey breast
	1	slice reduced fat cheese
		mustard
	4	vanilla wafers
SNACK	1/4	of a cantaloupe
DINNER	1	baked chicken breast
	1/2	cup rice
	1	cup cooked carrots
SNACK	1	cup low fat yogurt

Day 2

BREAKFAST	1 bowl of cream of wheat 1 piece of dry toast, spread with apple sauce 1 cup skim milk
SNACK	1 boiled egg
LUNCH	1 1/2 cup *Tuna Casserole* 1 roll 1/2 cup frozen yogurt
SNACK	1 banana
DINNER	1 Stuffed Baked Potato* green beans 1 baked apple
SNACK	4 vanilla wafers

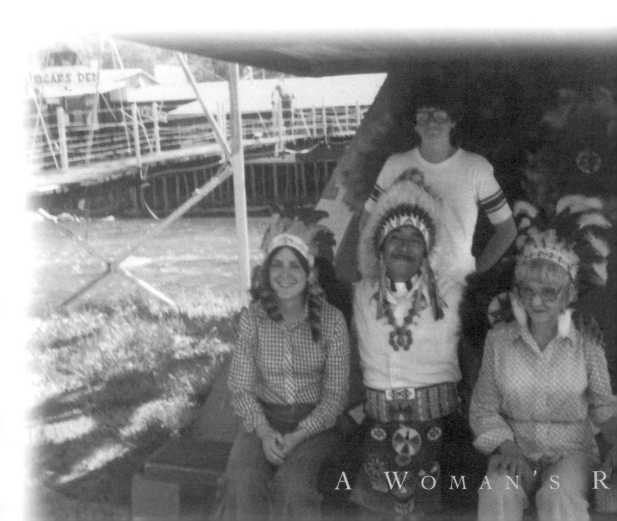

A WOMAN'S R

Day 3

BREAKFAST 3/4 cup puffed rice cereal
1 cup skim milk
1 banana

SNACK 3 graham cracker squares

LUNCH 1 large bowl Chicken and Vegetable
Soup*
6 saltine crackers
1/2 cup seedless grapes

SNACK 1/4 of a cantaloupe

DINNER 1 cup *Chicken and Potato Bake*
green peas
1 roll
1 cup pudding, made with skim milk

SNACK 1 pear

He that is of a merry heart hath a continual feast.

– Proverbs 15:15

There are elements so diverse that they cannot be joined in the heart of man.

– *Jean Giraudoux*

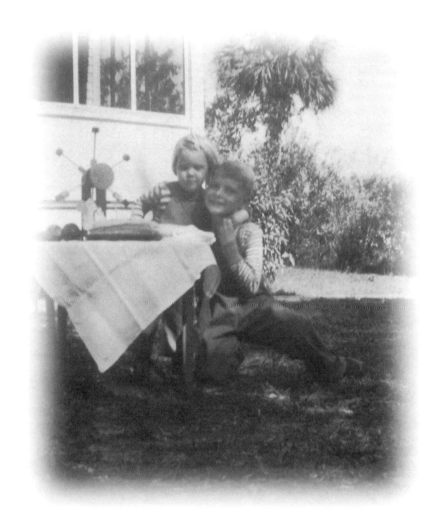

DAY 4

BREAKFAST	1 bowl of cream of wheat 1 banana 1 cup skim milk
SNACK	3 graham crackers
LUNCH	*Turkey and Pasta Salad* 1 cup applesauce 1 roll
SNACK	1/2 cup frozen yogurt
DINNER	1 6-ounce portion baked fish 1/2 cup rice summer squash, cooked with onion (optional)
SNACK	4 vanilla wafers

DAY 5

BREAKFAST	1 boiled egg 1 bagel all-fruit jam
SNACK	1 pear
LUNCH	2 slices whole wheat bread 1 to 2 slices turkey breast 1 slice reduced fat cheese mustard 1 cup applesauce
SNACK	3 graham crackers
DINNER	1 broiled, boneless pork loin chop (all visible fat removed) 1 cup Healthy Mashed Potatoes* cooked carrots 1 roll
SNACK	1/2 cup low fat yogurt

Day 6

BREAKFAST	3/4 cup puffed rice cereal
	1 cup skim milk
	1 banana
SNACK	3 graham crackers
LUNCH	Cooked vegetable plate:
	green beans, carrots, summer squash
	1 cup rice
SNACK	1 cup skim milk
DINNER	1 6-ounce portion baked fish
	1/2 cup Low Fat Macaroni and Cheese*
	green peas
	1 roll
SNACK	1 pear

Day 7

BREAKFAST	1 egg , scrambled in Pam
	1 slice whole wheat toast
	1/4 of a cantaloupe
	1 cup skim milk
SNACK	1/2 cup seedless grapes
LUNCH	2 slices whole wheat bread
	1/2 cup Terrific Tuna Salad*
	1 cup applesauce
	4 vanilla wafers
SNACK	1 cup skim milk
DINNER	1 baked or grilled chicken breast,
	all visible fat removed before
	cooking
	1 cup Low Fat Scalloped Potatoes
	green beans
SNACK	1/2 cup low fat frozen yogurt

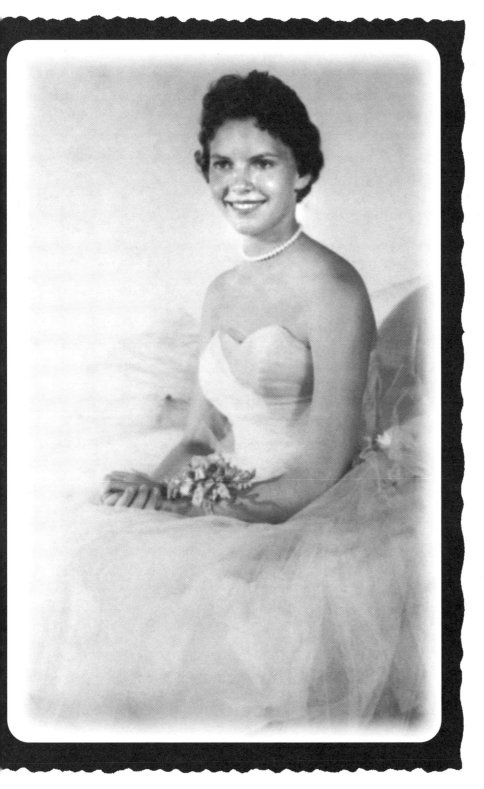

A thing of beauty is a joy forever, Its loveliness increases; it will never Pass into nothingness.

– *Keats*

TUNA CASSEROLE

1 can of water-packed tuna, drained
1 can English peas, drained
1 can reduced-fat cream of mushroom soup
8 ounces of pasta, cooked and drained
3/4 cup skim milk
    bread crumbs
    buttery flavored non-stick spray

Combine tuna, peas, soup, pasta, and milk.
Add salt and pepper to taste.
Pour into a casserole coated with non-stick spray.
Top with bread crumbs, then spray lightly with non-stick spray.
Bake at 350 degrees for 30 minutes.

CHICKEN / POTATO BAKE

2 chicken breasts, skin removed
2 baking potatoes, scrubbed and thinly sliced
1 onion, sliced into thin rings
2 carrots, thinly sliced
  salt and pepper
2 pieces of aluminum foil

Place 1 chicken breast on each piece of foil.
Place potato slices, onion, carrots, and salt/pepper on each breast.
Seal tightly and bake at 350 degrees for 1 hour.

Turkey Pasta Salad

1 cup cooked turkey breast, cut into chunks
8 ounces pasta, cooked and cooled
1 package frozen snow peas, cooked and cooled
1 can mushrooms, drained
1 cup low fat mozzarella cheese, cubed
1 Tablespoon reduced fat mayonnaise
2 Tablespoons Honey Mustard Dressing*

Combine all ingredients.
Toss lightly. Keep refrigerated until served.

Low Fat Scalloped Potatoes

4 potatoes, scrubbed and thinly sliced
2 onions, sliced into thin rings
1 can evaporated skim milk
4 Tablespoons all-purpose flour
2 Tablespoons reduced calorie margarine

Layer potatoes and onions, sprinkling with flour between the layers.
Pour skim milk over all. Dot with margarine.
Bake at 425 degrees for 1 to 1 1/2 hours.

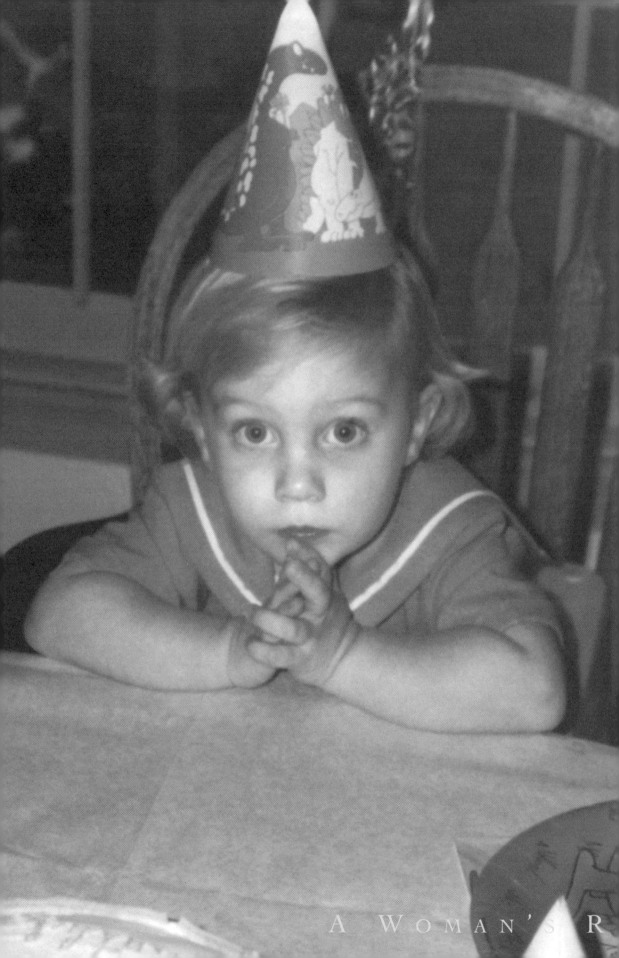

Frozen Yogurt Pie

1 box chocolate graham cookies, crushed
2 Tablespoons margarine, melted
2 8-ounce containers low fat flavored yogurt
1 8 ounce container light whipped topping
   fresh fruit

   Combine crushed cookies and margarine, mix well.
   Press into 8-inch square pan.
   Bake at 350 degrees for 5 minutes, cool.
   Combine yogurt and whipped topping, blending well.
   Pour yogurt mixture on top of cookie crust.
   Freeze. Slice to serve, and garnish with fresh fruit.(Match the fruit to the
   flavor of yogurt selected.)

Yields: 8 servings; calories: 334; total fat: 15g; saturated fat: 8g; cholesterol: 1mg;
sodium: 289mg; carbohydrates: 45g; calcium: 45mg; iron: 0mg.

Mom's Goodies

8 ounces lite sour cream
8 ounces low fat whipped topping
1 20-ounce can crushed pineapple, drained
1 11-ounce can mandarin oranges, chopped
1/2 cup pecans, chopped
6 to 8 maraschino cherries, chopped
1 Tablespoon cherry juice

   Blend sugar and sour cream, stir in remaining ingredients.
   Spoon into cupcake liners in muffin tin, freeze, and use as needed.

Yields: 12 servings; calories: 182; total fat: 10g; saturated fat: 6g; cholesterol: 6mg;
sodium: 15mg; carbohydrates: 21g; calcium: 34mg; iron: 0mg.

APPLE CRUMB CAKE

4 apples, sliced
  buttery flavored non-stick spray
1/2 cup brown sugar
1/4 cup all-purpose flour
1/4 cup rolled oats
1 teaspoon cinnamon
2 Tablespoons sugar
2 Tablespoons reduced calorie margarine

Place apples in square pan, coated with non-stick spray.
Spray tops of apples with buttery spray.
Combine brown sugar, flour, rolled oats, cinnamon, and sugar.
Cut in margarine. Sprinkle over top of apples.
Bake at 350 minutes for 30 minutes.

Yields: 8 servings; calories:128; total fat: 2g; saturated fat: 0g; cholesterol: 0mg;
sodium: 21mg; carbohydrates: 27g; calcium: 19mg; iron: 1mg.

FRUIT SHORTCAKE

1 angel food cake
2 cups fresh berries (strawberries, raspberries, blackberries, or blueberries)
1 8-ounce container of whipped topping

Slice cake into 1-inch slices.
Cover each slice with berries; top with 2 Tablespoons of whipped topping.

Yields: 12 servings; calories: 215; total fat: 5g; saturated fat: 5g; cholesterol: 0mg;
sodium: 397mg; carbohydrates: 37g; calcium: 78mg; iron: 0mg.

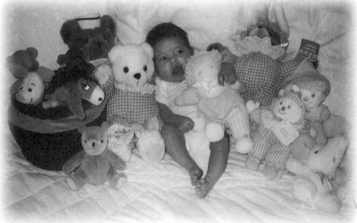

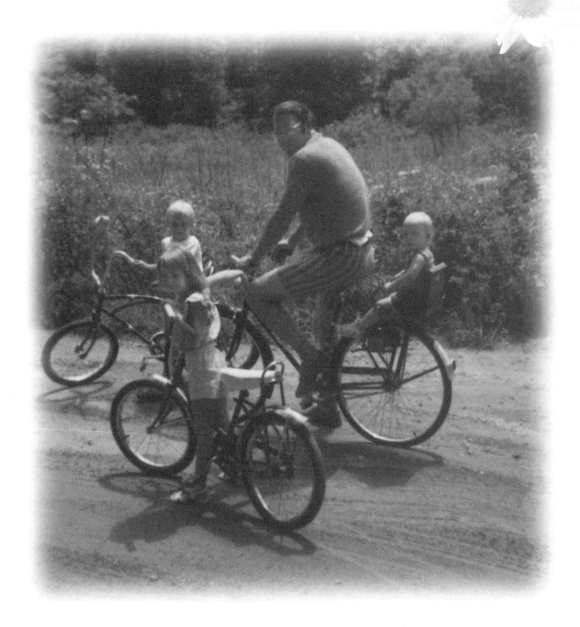

There is the difference between happiness and wisdom; he that thinks himself the happiest man really is so; but he that thinks himself the wisest, is generally the greatest fool.

– Colton

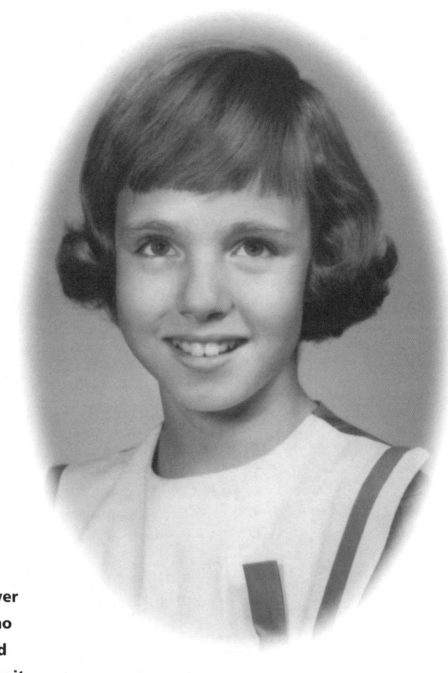

He who receives a good turn should never forget it; he who does one should never remember it.

– Charron

SWEET POTATO PIE

1   can sweet potatoes, drained and mashed
1/2   cup margarine, softened
1 1/2 cups sugar
1   Tablespoon flour
1   teaspoon vanilla
6   egg whites
1   can evaporated skim milk

Beat together potatoes, sugar, flour, and vanilla.
Add egg whites, beat well.
Add evaporated skim milk, beat well.
Pour into unbaked, deep dish pie crust.
Bake at 350 degrees for 45 minutes, or until center is set.

Yields: 8 servings; calories: 318; total fat: 12g; saturated fat: 3g; cholesterol: 2mg;
sodium: 218mg; carbohydrates: 50g; calcium: 107mg; iron: 1mg.

COCONUT PIE

1 1/2 cups sugar
4   egg whites
1/2 teaspoon salt
1/2 cup margarine, softened
1/4 cup flour
1/2 cup skim milk
1 1/2   cups coconut

Beat together sugar, egg whites, and salt.
Add margarine and flour, mix well.
Stir in milk and coconut.
Pour into unbaked deep dish pie crust.
Bake at 325 degrees for 1 hour.

Yields: 8 servings; calories: 374; total fat: 20g; saturated fat: 10g; cholesterol: 1mg;
sodium: 279mg; carbohydrates: 46g; calcium: 28mg; iron: 1mg

Variation:
Substitute 1 cup coconut, 1/2 cup crushed pineapple, drained, and 1/2 cup
almonds for the 1 1/2 cups coconut.

RECIPE INDEX

APPETIZERS

BREADS

DESSERTS

MAIN DISHES

SALADS

SIDE DISHES

Soups

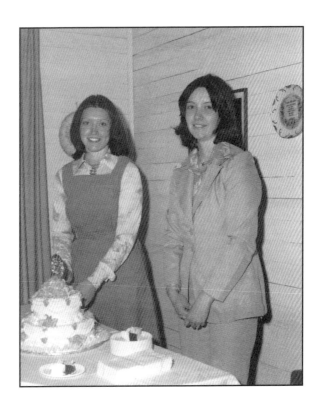